SpringerBriefs in Computer Science

Series Editors
Stan Zdonik

Shashi Shekhar

Jonathan Katz

Xindong Wu

Lakhmi C. Jain

David Padua

Xuemin (Sherman) Shen

Borko Furht

V.S. Subrahmanian

Martial Hebert

Katsushi Ikeuchi

Bruno Siciliano

Sushil Jajodia

Newton Lee

More information about this series at http://www.springer.com/series/10028

Sriraam Natarajan • Kristian Kersting
Tushar Khot • Jude Shavlik

Boosted Statistical Relational Learners

From Benchmarks to Data-Driven Medicine

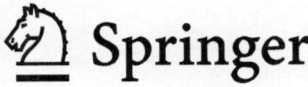 Springer

Sriraam Natarajan
Indiana University
Bloomington, Indiana
USA

Kristian Kersting
TU Dortmund University
Dortmund
Germany

Tushar Khot
Indiana University
Bloomington, Indiana
USA

Jude Shavlik
University of Wisconsin
Madison, Wisconsin
USA

ISSN 2191-5768   ISSN 2191-5776 (electronic)
SpringerBriefs in Computer Science
ISBN 978-3-319-13643-1   ISBN 978-3-319-13644-8 (eBook)
DOI 10.1007/978-3-319-13644-8

Library of Congress Control Number: 2014960238

Springer Cham Heidelberg New York Dordrecht London

Printed on acid-free paper

Springer is part of Springer Science+Business Media (www.springer.com)

Acknowledgements

We gratefully acknowledge the contributions of all the co-authors of the several papers written on this topic. Specifically, we are thankful to Bernd Guttmann, Prasad Tadepalli, Saket Joshi, Gautam Kunapuli, Phillip Odom, Jeremy Weiss, David Page, Jose Picado, Baidya Saha, Adam Edwards, Chris Whitlow, Joe Maldjian, Jeff Carr for their contributions and discussions on several topics in this research.

Sriraam Natarajan, Jude Shavlik and Tushar Khot acknowledge DARPA Machine Reading Program and Deep Exploration and Filtering of Text Program under the Air Force Research Laboratory (AFRL) prime contract no. FA8750-09-C-0181 and FA8750-13-2-0039 respectively. Kristian Kersting's research leading to this monograph was partly supported by the Fraunhofer ATTRACT fellowship STREAM and by the European Commission under contract number FP7-248258-First-MM.

Contents

Chapter 1
Introduction

There is no doubt the role of structure and relations within data becomes more and more important nowadays—for example, Google, Facebook, world wide mind etc. In many learning and mining tasks information about one objects can help a learner to reach conclusions about other, related objects and in turn to improve its overall performance. However, relations are difficult to represent using a fixed set of propositional features i.e., vectors of fixed dimensions—the standard approach within statistical machine learning and data mining. To overcome this, Statistical Relational Learning (SRL) Getoor and Taskar (2007) studies the combination of relational learning (e.g. inductive logic programming) and statistical machine learning. By combining the power of logic and probability, such approaches can perform robust and accurate reasoning and learning about complex relational data. The advantage of these formulations is that they can succinctly represent probabilistic dependencies among the attributes of different related objects, leading to a compact representation of learned models. Most of these methods essentially use first-order logic to capture domain knowledge and soften the rules using probabilities or weights. These approaches range can be broadly classified into directed models (Getoor et al. 2001; Heckerman et al. 2004; Jaeger 1997; Kersting and De Raedt 2007; Milch et al. 2004; Neville and Jensen 2007; Ngo and Haddawy 1995; Poole 1993; Sato and Kameya 2001) and undirected models (Domingos and Lowd 2009; Gutmann and Kersting 2006; Taskar et al. 2002). The advantage of these models is that they can succinctly represent probabilistic dependencies among the attributes of different related objects, leading to a compact representation of learned models.

While statistical relational models are indeed highly attractive due to their compactness and comprehensibility, learning them is typically much more demanding than learning propositional ones. Most of these methods essentially use first-order logic to capture domain knowledge and soften the rules using probabilities or weights. At least this was the goal of the models that were developed initially in this area. This is due to the fact that Inductive Logic Programming (Muggleton and Raedt 1994) as a field was evolving then. This field concerns mainly with the problem of learning first-order rules from data. So early systems simply used a logic learner underneath to learn the rules and simply employed probabilistic learning techniques such as maximum likelihood estimation (for complete data) and EM (for incomplete data) to

© The Author(s) 2014
S. Natarajan et al., *Boosted Statistical Relational Learners*,
SpringerBriefs in Computer Science, DOI 10.1007/978-3-319-13644-8_1

Fig. 1.1 Trade-offs between
expert's time and learning
time for learning problems in
SRL models

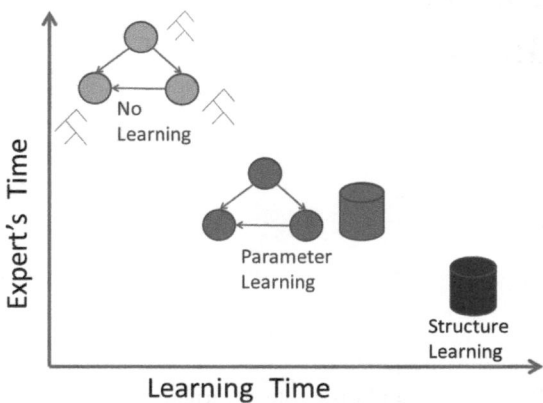

learn the parameters (i.e., weights or probabilities) for these rules. This is due to the
fact learning structure of a SRL model requires learning the parameters repeatedly
in the inner loop which in turn can sometimes require probabilistic inference in its
inner loop. This problem is exaggerated for SRL models since the predicates can
allow for arbitrary combinations of variables or constants as arguments[1].

To summarize, many early SRL methods rely on the structure as well as the
parameters of the models being specified by an expert. With the availability of training
data, it became possible to learn the parameters of the model using training data while
using the structure defined from the expert.

Parameter learning reduced the amount of effort needed from the expert and
potentially improved the accuracy of the model (by relying on data to correct mistakes
made by experts), but also increased the computational time. For some domains, the
structure of the model may be non-trivial, not known or insufficient. As a result, both
the structure and parameters of the model need to be learned from the data.

Although *structure learning* reduces the expert's effort, it can be computationally
intensive due to the large space of possible structures while including parameter
learning as a sub-task. Figure 1.1 shows this trade-off between the computation cost
and expert's effort. This book focuses on reducing the learning time while improving
the accuracy of structure learning in SRL models.

So, is scaling up learning of SRL models insurmountable? No, as we will argue
here. Typical SRL approaches seek to learn a single best SRL model. However, if
learning a single best and easy-to-interpret model is difficult, we should maybe stop
acting as if our goal is to do so, and instead embrace (model) complexity: we turn the
problem of learning a single SRL model into a series of relational regression problems

---

[1] For instance, when learning to predict if someone (say x) is popular, it is possible to use the predicate *Friends* in several ways. Some possible ways are *Friends(x,y)*, *Friends(y,x)*, *Friends(x, "Erdos")*
and *Friends("Erdos",x)*. Of course, the constant "Erdos" can be replaced with all possible constants
in the data base.

learned in a stage-wise manner using Friedman's functional gradient boosting Friedman (2001). This is a sensible idea since finding many rough rules of thumb of how to change a model can be a lot easier than finding a single model.

Specifically, the book presents a non-parametric approach to learning SRL models. The key idea is to turn the problem of learning relational probabilities as a series of relational regression problems. Specifically, triggered by the intuition that finding many rough rules of thumb of how to change one's probabilistic predictions locally can be a lot easier than finding a single, highly accurate model, we turned the problem of learning SRL models (bi-directed and undirected models) into a series of relational function approximation problems using gradient-based boosting. Specifically, we applied Friedman's (2001) gradient boosting to SRL models. That is, we represent each conditional probability distribution in a dependency network as a weighted sum of regression models that are grown via a stage-wise optimization. This extension allows for the algorithm to be adapted to different types of SRL models as we will discuss in the book. More importantly, this generalizable nature of the algorithm allows for it to be applied to several real world tasks such as heart attack prediction, Alzheimer's prediction, natural language processing tasks, real time strategy games etc. We discuss these applications and present the details of the adaptation of the algorithm to these domains.

Organization of the Book
The book is organized as follows: We present the required background for the book in Chap. 2 where we survey the area of SRL briefly and present the current learning methods in this area. We also introduce the domains that we will use for empirical evaluation throughout the book. We then consider one type of SRL model namely the bi-directed Relational Dependency Network and present the algorithm of gradient boosting as applied to this model. This is then extended to un-directed Markov Logic Network case in Chap. 4. In Chap. 5, we adapt these two algorithms to the case of missing data and show how both bi-directed and undirected models can be learned this way. Finally, in Chap. 6 we introduce the application and adaptation of these ideas to related tasks before concluding the book with some directions for future research.

Chapter 2
Statistical Relational Learning

This chapter presents background on SRL models on which our work is based on. We start with a brief technical background on first-order logic and graphical models. In Sect. 2.2, we present an overview of SRL models followed by details on two popular SRL models. We then present the learning challenges in these models and the approaches taken to solve them in literature. In Sect. 2.3.3, we present functional-gradient boosting, an ensemble approach[1], which forms the basis of our learning approaches. Finally, We present details about the evaluation metrics and datasets we used.

2.1 Representing Structure and Uncertainty

We first define some notation that is used throughout this book. We use capital letters such as X, Y, Z to represent variables and small letters such as x, y, z to represent values taken by the variables. We use bold-faced letters to represents sets. Letters such as $\mathbf{X}, \mathbf{Y}, \mathbf{Z}$ represent sets of variables and $\mathbf{x}, \mathbf{y}, \mathbf{z}$ represent sets of values. We use $\mathbf{z}_{-z}$ to denote $\mathbf{z}\backslash z$, i.e., every element from $\mathbf{z}$ except z. Similarly $\mathbf{x}_{-i}$ is used to represent $\mathbf{x}\backslash x_i$.

2.1.1 Representation: First-Order Logic

A simplistic view of first-order logic (FOL) is that it generalizes propositional logic by introducing variables as arguments to propositions (p to $p(\mathsf{X})$) which can be used to make logical statements about all objects in the domain (Russell and Norvig 2003). To avoid confusion with random variables, We use sans-serif capital letters X, Y, and Z

---

[1] Ensemble methods learn multiple models instead of one Bishop (2006).

© The Author(s) 2014
S. Natarajan et al., *Boosted Statistical Relational Learners*,
SpringerBriefs in Computer Science, DOI 10.1007/978-3-319-13644-8_2

Table 2.1 First-order logic terminology

Constants	Represent objects in the domain
	E.g., *anna, bob*
Variables	A variable can be assigned a value from a range of constants
	E.g., Variable X may take a value from $\{anna, bob\}$.
Predicate	Represents relations between objects in the domain
	E.g., the *Friends* predicate captures the friendship relation
Atom	A predicate along with its arguments
	E.g., $Friends(X,Y)$, $Father(bob, anna)$
Literal	An atom or its negation
	E.g., $Friends(anna, bob)$, $\neg Father(\mathsf{X},\mathsf{Y})$
Grounding	Substituting a variable with a constant
	E.g., A possible grounding of $Father(\mathsf{X},\mathsf{Y})$ is $Father(bob, anna)$
Ground atom/literal	An atom/literal without any variables E.g., $Friend(bob, anna)$
Clause	A disjunction (i.e., OR) of literals E.g., $Friend(\mathsf{X},\mathsf{Y}) \vee Father(\mathsf{X},\mathsf{Y})$ states that either X is a friend of Y *OR* X is the father of Y
Horn clause	A clause with only one positive literal commonly represented with an implication ($Body \Rightarrow Head$) having one literal in the head E.g., $Friend(\mathsf{X},\mathsf{Y}) \wedge Smokes(\mathsf{Y}) \Rightarrow Smokes(\mathsf{X})$, i.e., $\neg Friend(\mathsf{X},\mathsf{Y}) \vee \neg Smokes(\mathsf{Y}) \vee Smokes(\mathsf{X})$

to represent logical variables. We use lower-case sans-serif letters such as x, y and z to represent values taken by logical variables i.e. objects in the domain. The common logical operators/quantifiers are $\wedge$ (AND), $\vee$ (OR), $\Rightarrow$ (implication—condition implies consequence), $\forall$ (for all) and $\exists$ (existential 0 true for at least one value). used in this book are:

Furthermore, we assume that all logical variables are implicitly universally quantified (i.e. $\forall$) unless explicitly existentially quantified. Table 2.1 presents sample definitions of first-order logic terms that are used in the book.

2.1.2   Uncertainty: Graphical Models

Graphical models (Koller and Friedman 2009) represent conditional dependence among random variables which can then be used to factor the joint distribution over these variables. The factored distribution also reduces the number of parameters needed to model the joint distribution. Undirected models such as Markov networks (Kindermann and Snell 1980) factor the joint distribution as the product over potentials defined over cliques in the graph (subject to a normalization term). The potentials are generally represented using the function ϕ and the normalization term using Z. Directed models such as Bayesian networks (Pearl 1988) represent the joint

Fig. 2.1 Different areas of AI
with respect to learning,
representation and uncertainty

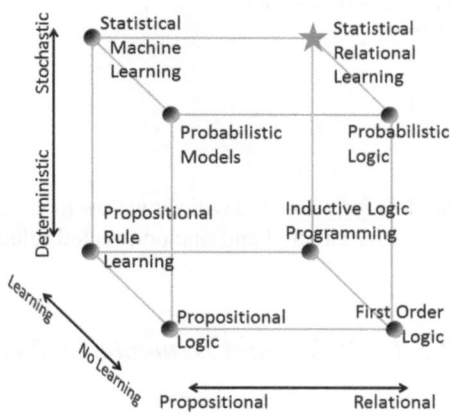

distributions as a product of conditional distributions for each variable given the parents of the variable. To ensure the product of conditional distributions represents the joint distribution, directed models require the model to be acyclic. The key idea is that the factored distributions can have exponentially smaller number of parameters compared to the full joint distribution.

Dependency networks (Heckerman et al. 2001) are directed graphical models that remove this acyclicity condition thereby allowing for faster learning of these models. But the product of the conditional distributions may not produce a consistent joint distribution.

2.2   Statistical Relational Models

Statistical Relational Learning (SRL) (Getoor and Taskar 2007) addresses the challenge of applying statistical inference and learning approaches to problems which involve rich collections of objects linked together in a complex, stochastic, and relational world. Figure 2.1 presents different areas in AI with respect to three dimensions: learning, representation and uncertainty. As can be observed, SRL extends statistical machine learning (Mitchell 1997) by using a richer representation, extends inductive logic programming (Lavrac and Dzeroski 1994; Raedt 2008) by modeling uncertainty and extends probabilistic logic (Nilsson 1986) by employing learning algorithms. The advantage of SRL models (Getoor et al. 2001; Heckerman et al. 2004; Jaeger 1997; Kersting and De Raedt 2007; Milch et al. 2004; Neville and Jensen 2007; Ngo and Haddawy 1995; Poole 1993; Sato and Kameya 2001; Domingos and Lowd 2009; Gutmann and Kersting 2006; Taskar et al. 2002) is that they can succinctly represent probabilistic dependencies among the attributes of different related objects, leading to a compact representation of learned models. We present two SRL

Fig. 2.2 A dependency
network

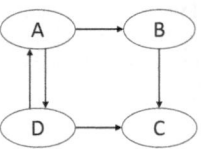

models for which we will show how to use boosting to learn them automatically from
data: one directed and one undirected relational model.

2.2.1 Relational Dependency Networks

Dependency networks (DNs) Heckerman et al (2001) are graphical models that approximate a joint probability distribution as a product of conditional probability
distributions (CPDs) $(P(\mathbf{X}) \approx \prod_i P(X_i \mid Pa(X_i)))$. Unlike Bayesian Networks, DNs
allow cycles in the graphical model, as a result the joint distribution is approximated. The key advantage of this approximation is that each conditional
distribution can be learned independently, which makes learning DNs much faster.
Figure 2.2 shows a sample DN where $P(A, B, C, D)$ is approximated by the product
$P(B|A)P(C|B, D)P(D|A)P(A|D)$. While these are approximate models, Heckerman et al. (2001) have shown that *ordered pseudo-Gibbs sampling* can be used to
recover the full joint distribution from these conditional distributions as long as each
conditional distribution is consistent.

Relational Dependency Networks (RDNs) are relational extensions of DNs. RDNs
are dependency networks where each node is a (first-order) predicate and the CPDs
capture the conditional distribution of a predicate given a subset of all the other
predicates. Similar to DNs, the network in RDNs can have cycles and hence approximate the joint distribution. Each predicate has an associated CPD conditioned on
the value of its parents. Each CPD can be compactly represented using models such
as Relational Probability Trees (RPT) (Neville et al. 2003a) or Relational Bayesian
Classifiers (RBC) (Neville et al. 2003b).

An example RDN is presented in Fig. 2.3 for an university domain. The ovals
indicate predicates, while the dotted boxes represent the objects in the domain. As
can be seen, there are *professor*, *student* and *course* objects with *taughtBy* and *takes*
as the relations among them. The nodes *avgSGrade* and *avgCGrade* are aggregator
functions over grades on students and courses respectively. The arrows indicate the
probabilistic (or possibly deterministic) dependencies among the predicates. For
example, the predicate *grade* has *difficulty*, *takes*, and *IQ* as its parents. Also note
that there is a bidirectional relationship between *satisfaction* and *takes*. Given the
structure along with the conditional distributions, we can now use ordered pseudo-
Gibbs sampling (Heckerman et al. 2001) to answer queries such as satisfaction of a
student.

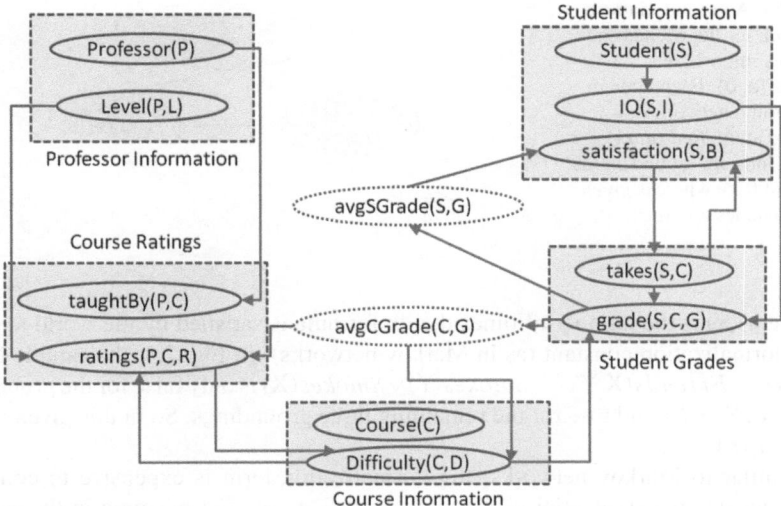

Fig. 2.3 A relational dependency network

2.2.2   Markov Logic Networks

Markov Logic Networks (MLNs) (Domingos and Lowd 2009) are relational models represented using weighted first-order logic rules. These rules provide a template for generating a Markov network by grounding the variables to all the constants[2] in the first-order logic rules. Each rule r_i forms a clique in the ground network and its weight w_i determine the potential for each clique. Fig. 2.4.

$$\text{Weight} = 1.1 \ \textit{Friends}(\mathsf{X,Y}) \wedge \textit{Smokes}(\mathsf{Y}) \rightarrow \textit{Smokes}(\mathsf{X})$$

This rule presents a MLN clause from a simple cancer domain (adopted from Domingos and Lowd 2009). The corresponding ground Markov network generated from this rule for a domain with two constants $\mathsf{X,Y} \in \{\mathsf{a,b}\}$ is shown in Fig. 2.4.

The joint probability distribution in a MLN is given by the product of the potentials on each clique, similar to Markov networks. For a given world state (truth value assignment to all ground atoms), the clique potential function returns e^{w_i} if the ground clause is true, otherwise it returns 1. Since all the cliques generated by grounding the same clause have the same weight, the probability of a given world state can be calculated using the number of true groundings of each clause. Hence the probability of the data is given by:

$$P(\mathbf{X} = \mathbf{x}) = \frac{1}{Z} \exp\left(\sum_i w_i n_i(\mathbf{x})\right)$$

---

[2] We assume a finite set of constants throughout this document.

Fig. 2.4 A ground Markov network for the friends and smokes rule where $X, Y \in \{a, b\}$. Each node in the ground network is a ground atom. *Red (dark)* nodes indicate ground atoms that are false whereas *green (light)* nodes are true

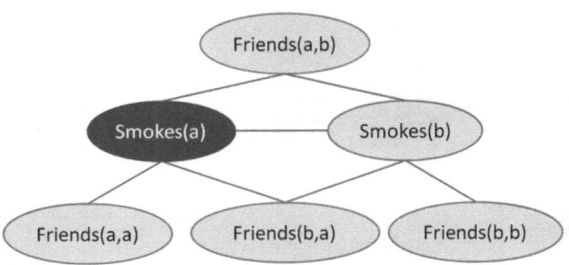

where $n_i(\mathbf{x})$ is the number of times the ith formula is satisfied by the world $\mathbf{x}$ and Z is a normalization constant (as in Markov networks). In Fig. 2.4, the sample MLN clause : $\neg Friends(X, Y) \vee \neg Smokes(Y) \vee Smokes(X)$ is only false for the grounding $\{X = a, Y = b\}$ and true for the remaining three groundings. So in this given world state, $n_i(\mathbf{x}) = 3$.

Similar to Markov networks, the normalization term is expensive to compute since its size is exponential in the number of features. For example in the sample MLN, the *Friends* predicate would have $O(n^2)$ groundings, where n is the number of people in the data set. Computation of the normalization terms requires summing over all these groundings. As a result, most learning methods use the approximate pseudo-likelihood (PL):

$$PL(\mathbf{X} = \mathbf{x}) = \prod_{X_i \in \mathbf{X}} P(X_i = x_i | MB(X_i))$$

where $MB(X_i)$ corresponds to the Markov blanket[3] of the ground atom, X_i in the ground Markov network. An avid reader must have noted that the pseudo-likelihood term is similar to the probability distribution of RDNs, which is also defined as a product of the conditional distributions.

2.3   Learning in SRL Models

SRL Models, and graphical models in general, are specified in terms of the *structure* of the model and the *parameters* defined over this structure. The structure defines the relations among the variables and the parameters quantify this relationship.

2.3.1   Parameter Learning

Since the parameters of a model are defined with respect to a model structure, the parameter-learning approaches assume that the structure is already provided.

---

[3] The Markov blanket of a node x_i is all the direct neighbors of x_i in the ground Markov network.

Directed Models
In case of directed models such as PRMs, BLPs and RDNs, it is assumed that the parents of every logical predicate is known. Similar to Bayesian networks, the problem of parameter learning in these models can be viewed as learning the conditional distributions for each predicate. The standard approach in this research is to formulate the optimization problem as either maximizing the log-likelihood or minimizing the mean squared error when given some training data (Natarajan et al. 2005; Natarajan et al. 2008; Kersting and De Raedt 2007; Getoor et al. 2001). Then either gradient-descent or EM algorithm is adapted to fill in the parameter values. Since relational models can have multiple instantations of a logical variable, either combining rules or aggregations are used to handle this issue. The algorithms are capable of learning the parameters of these combining rules as well.

Undirected Models
In MLNs, since the first-order logic rules specify the cliques in the network, the parameter-learning problem corresponds to learning the weights of the rules. The earliest approaches for learning the weights in MLNs used gradient descent (Singla and Domingos 2005) where the gradients for the weight of the clause are computed. The issue is that this gradient computation requires computation of the expected number of groundings of the clause which in turn requires inference at each step. So approximations such as maximum a posteriori (MAP) estimates were used instead of the actual expectation. This work was later extended to second-order gradient descent approach (Lowd and Domingos 2007) and to margin-based approaches (Huynh and Mooney 2009, 2011). But all of these approaches perform iterative updates to the weights where each update computation needs to perform inference. As a result, even parameter learning in MLNs can be computationally intensive.

2.3.2   Structure Learning

Unlike parameter learning, structure-learning approaches search over the space of possible structures for a model. Generally structure-learning approaches use a scoring function to evaluate a structure, a hypothesis space of valid structures to search over and a search strategy to search within the hypothesis space. Since the number of possible structures for relational models can be very large (structure learning is NP-Hard even in propositional models; Chickering 1996), most approaches use a greedy search strategy in the hypothesis space. Since the predictive performance of a structure (standard scoring function) depends on the parameters too, the search procedure needs to learn the parameters for every candidate structure, increasing the computational complexity of structure learning.

Most early structure learning methods employed the use of Inductive Logic Programming (ILP) (Muggleton and Raedt 1994) that learned logical theories such that these theories cover most of the positive examples and as few as possible of a set of negative examples. They perform a greedy search for the set of "clauses" that are consistent with the training examples. Needless to say that these are deterministic clauses which do not handle noisy data well. However, these are the early techniques that inspired several structure learning methods inside SRL. One successful adaptation of this inductive learning method is the learning of TILDE trees (Blockeel and Raedt 1998). These trees upgrade the attribute representation of the classical decision trees by allowing for logical clauses as tests inside each node. Hence, learning a decision tree can be understood as learning a decision list of first-order clauses using some ILP learning method. TILDE trees extend this learning by computing regression values (or probabilities) in the leaves of these trees. This is one of the earliest successful statistical relational structure learning method. We now present the other more recent methods briefly.

Directed Models

Most directed models such as BLPs and PRMs use a greedy hill-climbing approach based on operators over the structure similar to the structure-learning approaches for Bayesian networks. BLPs define operators such as adding or removing literals from clauses, replacing variables by constants or vice versa, and adding or removing clauses. PRMs, on the other hand, define a set of potential parents for every target attribute and only considers adding/removing a parent from this set during the greedy search. The commonality is that to score a candidate structure, both the models first calculate the parameters based on counts in the data as mentioned before. The candidate structure with the highest score (calculated based on the likelihood of the training data) is accepted and the process continues.

The simplest among all directed models is the case of local models such as RDNs where learning the set of conditional distributions independently is sufficient to learn the structure. Neville and Jensen (2007) use two models: Relational Probability Trees (RPT; Neville et al. 2003a) and Relational Bayesian Classifiers (RBC; Neville et al. 2003b) to model the conditional distributions. A simple way to understand this learning is that at the start of learning process, all the other predicates are assumed to be parents of the target predicate. Then learning corresponds to simply finding the best tree that models the conditional distribution (similar to feature selection in a decision tree for propositional machine learning). Hence, an RDN is a set of RPTs learned one after another.

Undirected Models

For undirected models, since most of the prior work as well as our work focuses on MLNs, we present structure-learning approaches for MLNs. Structure learning in MLNs corresponds to learning the clauses along with the weights of these clauses. The initial approach to learn MLN structure avoided learning parameters for every structure by learning the structure, i.e., the clauses of the model first and then learning the parameters (Richardson and Domingos 2004). They used CLAUDIEN (Van Laer et al. 1994), a first-order logic clause learner, to first learn the rules and then learned the weights of the rules. But this approach does not take the potential parameters into account before scoring the clauses and as a result can be sub-optimal. Following this work, Kok and Domingos (2005) developed a structure-learning approach that searched over the space of clauses and learned the weights for scoring each candidate structure. Bottom-up structure learning (Mihalkova and Mooney 2007) uses a propositional Markov network learning algorithm to identify paths of ground atoms. These form the templates that are generalized into first-order formulas. Hypergraph lifting (Kok and Domingos 2009) on the other hand clusters the constants and true atoms to construct a lifted (first-order) graph. Relational path-finding on this hypergraph is used to obtain the MLN clauses. Structural motif learning (Kok and Domingos 2010) uses random walks on the ground network to find symmetrical paths and cluster nodes with similar path distributions. All these methods obtain the candidate clauses first, learn the weights and modify the clauses.

2.3.3   *Functional-Gradient Boosting*

Recall from the introduction that the goal of this book is to bring the complexity of structure learning as close to parameter learning as possible. To this effect, we now present a learning algorithm that in the propositional case can learn the parameter and structure of the model simultaneously.

Most machine learning approaches use a parametric model that optimizes a specific loss function. For example, the logistic regression model uses a weight parameter w, and uses gradient descent to find the best parameters that maximize the likelihood of the data. Let $\{x_1, \ldots, x_n\}$ be the set of examples and $\{y_1, \ldots, y_n\}$ be their corresponding binary labels (represented as 1 and -1). In a logistic regression model, the probability of a label for a given example is given by $P(y_i|x_i; w) = 1/(1 + e^{-y_i w^T x_i})$. Assuming the examples are independent, the log-likelihood (LL) of the full dataset is given by

$$LL(\mathbf{y}, \mathbf{x}; w) = \sum_{x_i \in \mathbf{x}} \log P(y_i|x_i; w)$$

The standard method of learning in these models is based on gradient descent where the learning algorithm starts with initial parameters w_0 and computes the gradient of the log-likelihood (LL) function. The gradient during the mth iteration is given by

$$\Delta_m = \frac{\partial LL(\mathbf{y}, \mathbf{x}; w_{m-1})}{\partial w_{m-1}}$$

and the weight parameter at the end of m iterations is given by

$$w_m = w_0 + \Delta_1 + \ldots + \Delta_m$$

Friedman (2001) suggested that instead of using a parametric approach, apply the numeric optimization in the function space. For example, the probability of an example can be defined to be $P(y_i|x_i; \psi) = 1/(1 + e^{-y_i \psi(x_i)})$ and the gradients can be computed with respect to the function ψ. Similar to parametric gradient descent,

Table 2.2 Training data with
class label **c**

#	a	b	c
1	1	0	1
2	0	0	0
3	1	1	0

we start with an initial function ψ_0 and compute the gradients with respect to the
function ψ:

$$\Delta_m = E_{x,y}\left[\frac{\partial LL(y,x;\psi_{m-1})}{\partial \psi_{m-1}}\right]$$

The ψ function at the end of m iterations is given by

$$\psi_m = \psi_0 + \Delta_1 + \ldots + \Delta_m$$

Since we only have a finite set of examples, rather than computing the gradients over
the entire space of possible examples, Friedman suggests calculating the gradient
for each training example. The gradient for an example x_i is given by $\Delta_m(x_i) = \partial LL(\mathbf{y},\mathbf{x};\psi_{m-1})/\partial \psi_{m-1}(x_i)$. We can then fit a regression function, $\hat{h}(x_i)$ to these
gradients, $\Delta_m(x_i)$. Most functional-gradient approaches learn a regression tree to
represent $\hat{h}$ and minimize the least-square error:

$$\hat{h}_m = \arg\min_h \sum_{x_i}[h(x_i) - \Delta_m(x_i)]^2$$

Since we approximated the gradients (Δ_m) using a regression function ($\hat{h}_m$), the
potential function ψ after the mth iteration is given by:

$$\psi_m = \psi_0 + \hat{h}_1 + \ldots + \hat{h}_m$$

Standard boosting approach Freund and Schapire (1996) learns a sequence of models
where the weight on the examples (think importance of the examples) is updated
after every iteration to increase the weight on incorrectly classified examples. As a
result, every subsequent model attempts to correct the mistakes in the current model.
FGB also learns a sequence of models ($\hat{h}_i$ in this case) where every subsequent
model focuses on the incorrectly classified examples (due to the example's higher
regression values), hence the *boosting* in its name.

Consider the small dataset with three examples shown in Table 2.2 with two fea-
tures (a and b) and the class label c. If we assume $P(y_i = 1|x_i;\psi) = 1/(1+e^{-\psi(x_i)})$,
the gradients can be shown to be $\Delta_m(x) = We(y_i = \hat{y}_i) - P(y_i = \hat{y}_i|x_i;\psi_m)$, where
$We(y_i = \hat{y}_i)$ is the indicator function and $\hat{y}_i$ is the true label of x_i in the training data.
Let us assume the initial prior ψ_0 returns 0 for every example i.e., $\psi_0(x) = 0, \forall x$.
Given this initial prior, all the examples would have the predicted probability of
$P(y_i = 1|x_i;\psi_0) = 0.5$, based on the current model.

Table 2.3 Initial regression dataset

#	a	b	Δ_1
1	1	0	0.50
2	0	0	−0.50
3	1	1	−0.50

Table 2.4 Regression values after tree 1

#	a	b	Δ_2
1	1	0	0.50
2	0	0	−0.37
3	1	1	−0.50

Fig. 2.5 A sample model for predicting class label c after m iterations

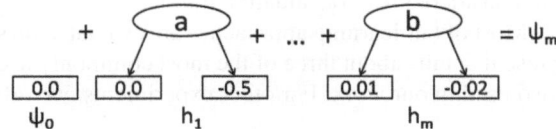

The gradient Δ for the positive example is 0.5 whereas for the negative examples is −0.5, as shown in Table 2.3. Hence the gradients for the positive examples are pushing the ψ function for those examples to a higher value, thereby pushing the predicted probability closer to 1. Let us assume that we learn a regression tree with only one node that tests for a being true or not. The left (true) branch would contain two examples (#1 and #3) and the right (false) branch would contain only one example (# 2). Since the mean of the regression values of examples #1 and #3 is zero, the left leaf would return zero. On the other hand, the right branch would return −0.50 as the regression value. So the learned regression function $\hat{h}_1$ to fit the Δ values shown in Table 2.3 is:

$$\hat{h}_1(x) = \quad 0.0 \qquad \text{if } a = 1$$
$$= -0.5 \qquad \text{if } a = 0$$

Since our ψ_0 function returned zero for all the examples, adding $\hat{h}_1$ to ψ_0 would give us $\psi_1 = \psi_0 + \hat{h}_1 = \hat{h}_1$ as our new current model. Given this model, we can compute the probabilities for the training examples. Since examples #1 and #3 have $\psi_1(x) = 0$, they still have the same gradients, but the gradient for example #2 has reduced to −0.37, as shown in Table 2.4. The next tree learned on this regression dataset would split on feature b and reduce the gradient on example #3, similar to what we observed in the previous step with example #2. Hence with each iteration, the gradients on the examples move closer to zero and our predicted probabilities would move closer to the observed values in the training data. Figure 2.5 shows a sample model ψ_m after m iterations of boosting.

2.4 Benchmark Datasets

We now present details about the evaluation approach used. To show that the boosting approach learns a more accurate model, we compare the accuracy of the probabilistic predictions made by the models using three evaluation measures commonly used in literature. In addition to conditional log-likelihood (CLL), we use the areas under Precision-Recall curve (AUC-PR) and Receiver Operating Characteristic curve (AUC-ROC) (Davis and Goadrich 2006). It has been shown that CLL is not a perfect measure when dealing with skewed data sets. Relational data is inherently skewed as most of the relations are generally false (the number of friends of a person is much smaller than the entire population). In such cases, AUC-PR and AUC-ROC are considered better evaluation metrics.

Most of our learning approaches are evaluated on standard SRL data sets. We will present details about three of the most commonly used data sets in literature that are also used in our work. For other experiments, we refer to the corresponding paper.

2.4.1 UW-CSE

The UW-CSE dataset (Richardson and Domingos 2006) was creating from University of Washington's Computer Science and Engineering department's student database (hence the name). The data set consists of details about professors, students and courses from five different sub-areas of computer science (AI, programming languages, theory, system and graphics). The dataset includes predicates such as *professor, student, publication, advisedBy, hasPosition, projectMember, yearsInProgram, courseLevel, taughtBy*, and *teachingAssistant* and equality predicates such as *samePerson, sameCourse* etc. The goal in this data set is to predict the *advisedBy* relationship between a student and a professor using the other predicates.

There are 4,106,841 possible *advisedBy* relations out of which 3380 relations are true. Since the dataset consists of five areas (or mega-examples), we performed five-fold cross-validation. Unless specified, we train on four areas and evaluated the results on the remaining area. This is the same approach taken in the MLN literature (Domingos and Lowd 2009) where each of the four areas form a "mega-example" that consists of all the inter-related objects of that area. Creating more folds would require breaking up the network of connected objects within each area. Hence each area is viewed as a single example. Our results are thus averaged over five mega-examples.

2.4.2 Cora

Cora dataset, now a standard dataset for citation matching, was first created by Andrew McCallum, and later segmented by Bilenko and Mooney (2003). The dataset was later converted into relational format by Poon and Domingos (2007). In citation matching, the task is to identify citations that refer to the same paper, which as a sub-task may include matching the author, title and venue of citations. A cluster is a set of citations that refer to the same paper, and a nontrivial cluster contains more than one citation. The Cora dataset has 1295 citations and 134 clusters where almost every citation in Cora belongs to a nontrivial cluster; the largest cluster contains 54 citations. Sets of clusters were combined to create five mega-examples by Poon and Domingos.

For each citation we have information about the various fields using predicates such as *author*, *title*, *venue*, *hasWordAuthor*, *hasWordTitle*, and *hasWordVenue*. This task has multiple target predicates (*sameAuthor*, *sameVenue*, *sameTitle*, and *sameBib*) for identifying matching authors, venues, titles and the complete citation. This dataset has five mega-examples and hence We perform 5-fold cross-validation to evaluate on this dataset.

2.4.3 IMDB

This dataset was created by Mihalkova and Mooney (2007) from IMDB.com and contains information about actors, movies, directors and the relationships between them. The predicates in this dataset are: *actor*, *director*, *workedUnder*, *genre*, and *gender*. The task is to predict the *workedUnder*, *genre*, and *gender* given all the other predicates. The *actor* and *director* predicates are mutually exclusive predicates (i.e., $actor(X) \Leftrightarrow \neg director(X)$) that provide type information for the people in the domain. Since the dataset is divided to five mega-examples by Mihalkova and Mooney (each mega-example contains four movies), we perform five-fold cross-validation in the experiments. Following Kok and Domingos (2009), we omitted the four equality predicates. The goal is to learn the conditional distribution to predict all the predicates except `actor` and `director`.

Chapter 3
Boosting (Bi-)Directed Relational Models

In this chapter, we show the use of functional gradient boosting for learning Relational Dependency Networks (RDNs). The use of several regression trees, instead of just one, results in an expressive model for the conditional distributions of RDNs. We then present a sample set of results that show superior performance when compared to state-of-the-art approaches.

3.1 Introduction

Recall that the main advantage of RDNs is that there are straightforward and computationally efficient algorithms for learning both the structure and probabilities of a dependency network from data. Essentially, the algorithm consists of independently performing a probabilistic classification or regression for each variable in the domain. Neville and Jensen (2007) to elegantly lift dependency networks to the relational case and employ relational probability trees for learning.

In this chapter, we describe a new learning approach for RDNs. Finding many rough rules of thumb of how to change our probabilistic predictions locally can be a lot easier than finding a single, highly accurate local model. Hence, we propose to apply Functional gradient boosting (Friedman 2001) to RDNs. That is, we represent each conditional probability distribution in a dependency network as a weighted sum of regression models grown in a stage-wise optimization. Such a functional gradient approach has recently been used to efficiently train conditional random fields for labeling (relational) sequences (Dietterich et al. 2004; Gutmann and Kersting 2006) and relational policies (Kersting and Driessens 2008).

The benefits of a boosting approach to RDNs are as follows: First, being a non-parametric approach the number of parameters can grow with the number of training episodes. In turn, interactions among random variables are introduced only as needed, so that the potentially infinite search space is not explicitly considered. Second, it is fast and easy to implement, at least when we have a relational regression tree learner at hand. Existing off-the-shelf regression learners can be used to deal with propositional, continuous, and relational domains in a unified way. Third, the use of

© The Author(s) 2014
S. Natarajan et al., *Boosted Statistical Relational Learners*,
SpringerBriefs in Computer Science, DOI 10.1007/978-3-319-13644-8_3

boosting for learning RDNs makes it possible to learn the structure and parameter simultaneously which is an attractive feature as structure learning in SRL models is computationally very expensive. Admittedly, we sacrifice comprehensibility for better predictive performance.

First, we present the basics of the learning algorithm and then followed by the empirical evaluations.

3.2   Boosting RDNs

As mentioned earlier, an RDN can be represented as a set of conditional distributions $P(Y|\mathbf{Pa}(Y))$ for all the predicates Y and learning RDNs correspond to learning the structure of these distributions along with their values. To employ functional gradient boosting, we use a functional representation of the parameters. This is to say that we consider the conditional distribution of a predicate, denoted simply for example as y_i to be

$$P(y_i|\mathbf{Pa}(y_i)) = e^{\psi(y_i;x_i)}/\sum_{y'} e^{\psi(y';x_i)} \forall x_i \in \mathbf{x}_i \neq y_i$$

where $\psi(y_i; x_i)$ is the potential function of y_i given all other predicates $x_i \neq y_i$. The gradient w.r.t the potential functions can be computed as:

$$P(y_i|\mathbf{x_i}) = \frac{e^{\psi(y_i;x_i)}}{\sum_{y'} e^{\psi(y';x_i)}} \Rightarrow log P(y_i|\mathbf{x_i}) = \psi(y_i;x_i) - log \sum_{y'} e^{\psi(y';x_i)}$$

$$\frac{\partial log P(y_i|\mathbf{x_i})}{\partial \psi(y_i = 1|\mathbf{x_i})} = I(y_i = 1; \mathbf{x_i}) - \frac{1}{\sum_{y'} e^{\psi(y';x_i)}} \frac{\partial \sum_{y'} e^{\psi(y';x_i)}}{\partial \psi(y_i = 1|\mathbf{x_i})}$$

$$= I(y_i = 1; x_i) - \frac{e^{\psi(y_i=1;x_i)}}{\sum_{y'} e^{\psi(y';x_i)}} = I(y_i = 1; \mathbf{x_i}) - P(y_i = 1; \mathbf{x_i})$$

In the above equation I is the indicator function. Note that as with the propositional case presented in the previous chapter, the new gradient is simply the adjustment required for the probabilities to match the observed value (y_i) in the training data for every example. Intuitively, this gradient is aiming to push all the predicates which are true in the world to a probability of 1 and the false predicates to a probability of 0. Also, it can be easily observed that the gradient of true target predicates is always ≥ 0 and the one for false target predicates is always ≤ 0.

This gradient serves as the weight for the current regression example at the next training episode. Following prior work (Gutmann and Kersting (2006), we use *relational regression trees* (Blockeel and Raedt 1998) to fit the gradient function at every position in the training example. An example is presented in Fig. 3.1**b**. The goal is to predict if A is *advisedBy* B. In the tree, if B is a *professor*, A is not a *professor*, A has more than one publication and more than one publication with B, then the regression

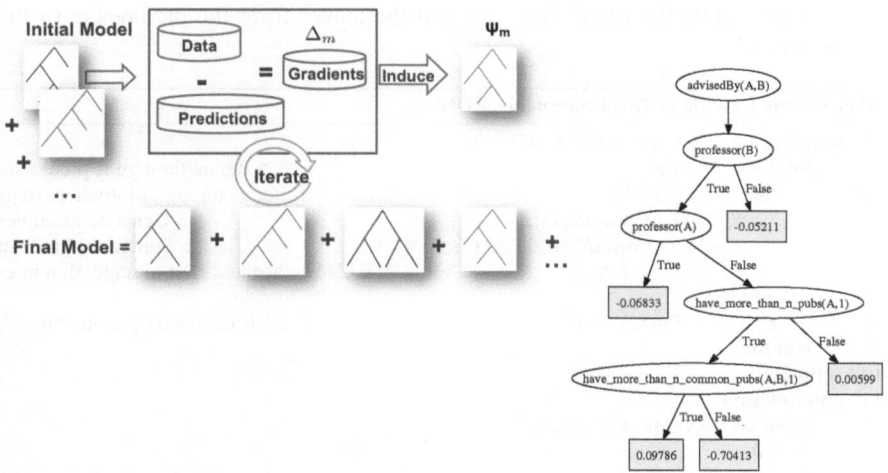

Fig. 3.1 **a** Example of an RDN. **b** Example of a relational regression tree

value is 0.09. As can be seen for most of the other cases, there are negative values indicating lower probabilities (< 0.5).

The key idea in this algorithm is to consider the conditional probability distribution of each predicate as a set of regression trees. These trees are learned such that at each iteration the new set of regression trees aim to maximize the likelihood of the distributions with respect to the potential function (see Fig. 3.1**a**).

When computing $P(a(X)|\mathbf{Pa}(a(X)))$ for a particular value of X (say x), each branch in each tree is considered to determine the branches that are satisfied and their corresponding regression values are added to the potential ψ. We use aggregators such as *count*, *max* and *average* to handle the case of multiple groundings of a predicate. We use the regression tree learner *TILDE* for learning the regression trees.

At a fairly high level, the learning of relational regression tree proceeds as follows: The learning algorithm starts with an empty tree and repeatedly searches for the best test for a node according to some splitting criterion such as weighted variance. Next, the examples in the node are split into success and failure according to the test. For each split, the procedure is recursively applied further obtaining subtrees for the splits. We use weighted variance on the examples as the test criterion. In our method, we use a small depth limit (of at most three) to terminate the search. In the leaves, the average regression values are computed.

The tree learner requires weighted examples as input where the weight of each example corresponds to the gradient presented above for the corresponding example. Note that the different regression trees provide the structure of the conditional distributions while the regression values at the leaves form the parameters of the distributions.[1]

Algorithm 1 Gradient Tree Boosting for RDN's

1: **function** TREEBOOSTFORRDNS(*Data*)
2:   **for** $1 \leq k \leq K$ **do**   ▷ Iterate through K predicates
3:     **for** $1 \leq m \leq M$ **do**   ▷ Iterate through M gradient steps
4:       $S_k := GenExamples(k; Data; F_{m-1}^k)$ ▷ Generate examples
5:       $\Delta_m(k) := FitRelRegressTree(S_k; L)$ ▷ Functional gradient
6:       $F_m^k := F_{m-1}^k + \Delta_m(k)$ ▷ Update Models - Set of regression trees
7:     **end for**
8:     $P(Y_k = y_k | \mathbf{Pa}(Y_k)) \propto \psi^k$ ▷ ψ^k is obtained by grounding F_M^k
9:   **end for**
10: **return**
11: **end function**
12: **function** GENEXAMPLES(*k, Data, F*)
13:   $S := \emptyset$
14:   **for** $1 \leq i \leq N_k$ **do**   ▷ Iterate over all examples
15:     Compute $P(y_k^i = 1 | \mathbf{Pa}(y_k^i))$ ▷ Probability of the predicate being true
16:     $\Delta(y_k^i) := I(y_k^i = 1) - P(y_k^i = 1 | \mathbf{Pa}(y_k^i))$ ▷ Compute Gradient
17:     $S := S \cup (y_k^i, \Delta(y_k^i))$ ▷ Update relational regression examples
18:   **end for**
19:   **return** S ▷ Return regression examples
20: **end function**

Our algorithm for learning RDNs using functional gradient is presented in Algorithm 3.2. Algorithm *TreeBoostForRDNs* is the main algorithm that iterates over all predicates. For each predicate (y_k), it generates the examples for the regression tree learner *TILDE* (that is called using function *FitRelRegressTree*) to get the new regression tree and updates its model (F_m^k). This is repeated for a pre-set number of iterations M (in our experiments, $M = 20$). Note that the after m steps, the current model F_m^k will have m regression trees each of which approximates the corresponding gradient for the predicate y_k. These regression trees serve as the individual components ($\Delta_m(k)$) of the final potential function.

The function *GenExamples* (line 4) is the function that generates the examples for *TILDE*. As can be seen, it takes as input the current predicate index (k), the data and the current model (F). The function iterates over all the examples and for each example, computes the probability and the gradient. Recall that for computing the probability of y_i, we consider all the trees learned for Y_i. For each tree, we compute the regression values based on the groundings of the current example. The gradient is then set as the weight of the example.

The algorithm *TreeBoostForRDNs* loops over all the predicates and learns the potentials for each predicate. The set of regression trees for each predicate forms the structure of the conditional distribution and the sets of leaves form the parameters of

---

[1] In reality, the values at the leaves form the gradients of parameters as there could be several possible regression trees for a given predicate.

Table 3.1 Results on UW data set

Algorithm	Likelihood	AUC-ROC	AUC-PR	Training Time
RDN-B	0.810	0.961	0.930	9 s
RDN	0.805	0.888	0.781	1 s
MLN	0.731	0.535	0.621	93 h

the conditional distribution. Thus gradient boosting allows us to learn the structure
and parameters of the RDN simultaneously.

3.3   Empirical Evaluation

We now present the results of evaluation on the three data sets that we presented in the
previous chapter. For more results and discussion, we refer the reader to Natarajan
et al. (2012b). We denote our learning algorithm as RDN-B (to make it clear that this
is RDN with Boosting and the adapted learning algorithm of Neville and Jensen that
uses a single relational tree as RDN.

3.3.1   UW Data Set

The results of the UW-dataset are presented in Table 3.1. We present the likelihood
on the test data ($\sum_i P(y_i = \hat{y}_i)$), the area under curve for PR and ROC[2] and the time
taken for training. As can be seen, *RDN-B* that use gradient tree boosting has the
best likelihood on the test data and is marginally (but statistically significantly) better
than the original RDN. MLNs on the other hand were able to identify the negative
examples but did not identify the positives well. For the AUC on both ROC and PR
curves, it is clear that *RDN-B* dominates all the other methods. For MLNs, we had to
use all the clauses that predicted *advisedBy* from the Alchemy website since learning
the structure on this data set was very expensive. Hence we learned only the weights
for these clauses and did not employ any structure learning algorithm. As can be
seen from the last column, weight learning for this data set took us 4 days as against
several seconds for our approach.

---

[2] We used http://mark.goadrich.com/programs/AUC/ to compute AUC.

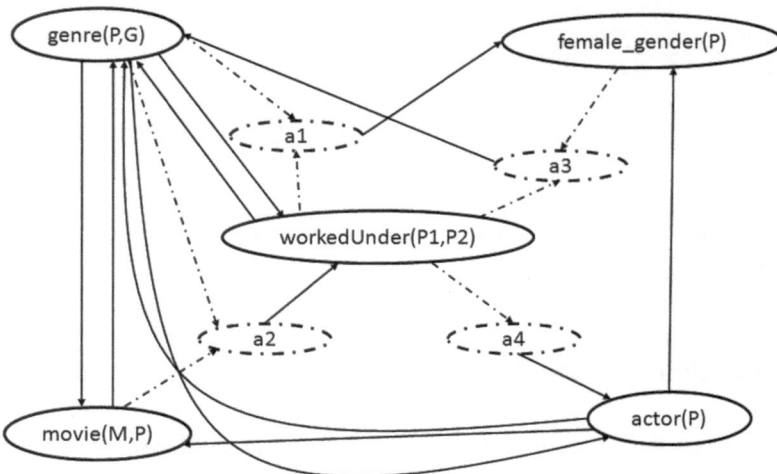

Fig. 3.2 RDN learned using boosting for the IMDB dataset. The *dashed nodes* are the aggregated nodes. For example, a_1 is an aggregation over *workedUnder* and *genre* predicates. For this model, all the nodes form the query predicates

3.3.2   IMDB Data Set

Before we present the results of the evaluation in this data set, we first present the learned structure. While in the previous data set, there was a single target relation. On the contrary, in this data set, we learn a joint model. We collected all the predicates present in the different trees for a particular target predicate and presented them in the figure. The dotted ovals are the aggregated predicates and there are four of them. a_1 is the aggregation performed over two predicates *genre* and *workedUnder*. Similarly, a_2 and a_3 are aggregations performed over *movie* and *genre* and *workedUnder* and *female_gender* predicates respectively. Note that a_4 is the aggregation over a single predicate *workedUnder*. Also, it is worth mentioning that unlike the original formulation of RDN that allow only for aggregated predicates to be in the model, we allow the original *non-aggregated* predicates as well. This is due to the fact that we treat the presence of these predicates as existentials, leading to more expressive models compared to original RDN models (Fig. 3.2).

The area under curve for precision-recall and ROC are presented in Fig. 3.3. The results are presented for three predicates *worked_under, genre,* and *female_gender*. We do not include predicates such as *actor, director* etc. for evaluation because they can be captured by mutual exclusivity rules and instead focused on the more interesting predicates. We have compared four different algorithms for this task. The algorithms compared are RDN-B that uses boosting, RDN learning that uses a single large regression tree and two different MLN learning algorithms BUSL (Mihalkova and Mooney 2007) and hypergraph lifting (Kok and Domingos 2009). The last two algorithms are shown as *BUSL* and *LHL* respectively in the figure. As

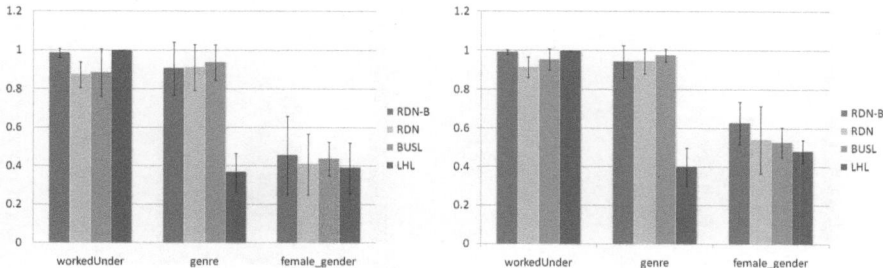

Fig. 3.3 Area under curves in IMDB dataset. The first graph shows the PR curve results while the second one is the area under curve for ROC curves

can be clearly seen, RDN-B performs consistently across all the query predicates. Hyper-graph lifting performs well for the *worked_under* but BUSL outperforms hyper-graph lifting in the other queries.

3.3.3 Cora Data Set

For this entity resolution task, the following predicates were used: author, title, venue, sameBib, sameAuthor, sameVenue, sameTitle, hasWordAuthor, hasWordTitle, hasWordVenue. We make a joint prediction over the predicates—SameBib, SameTitle, SameVenue and SameAuthor. We used the *B+N+C+T* MLN presented in Singla et al. (Singla and Domingos 2006) and available on the Alchemy website to compare against the boosted and non-boosted versions of RDN. Note that we are not learning the structure of MLN, but merely learn the weights of the MLN clauses. In the case of RDN and RDN-B, we learn the structure and parameters of the model.

The area under curves of the PR and ROC curves for the entity resolution task are presented in Fig. 3.4. The results are averaged over 5-folds for the four predicates that we mentioned earlier. As can be seen, RDN-B dominates the other methods consistently on all the four different predicates. MLNs exhibit good performance in the case of *SameAuthor* predicate, but are outperformed by the RDN methods in the other predicates. RDN learning that does not use boosting performs reasonably well, but is still outperformed by RDN-B in all the predicates in both the metrics.

3.4 Discussion

In summary, our experiments showed that the boosted version of RDN learning dominated the non-boosted version and the standard MLN learning methods in all the tasks. As mentioned earlier, these experiments are only a subset of the evaluation

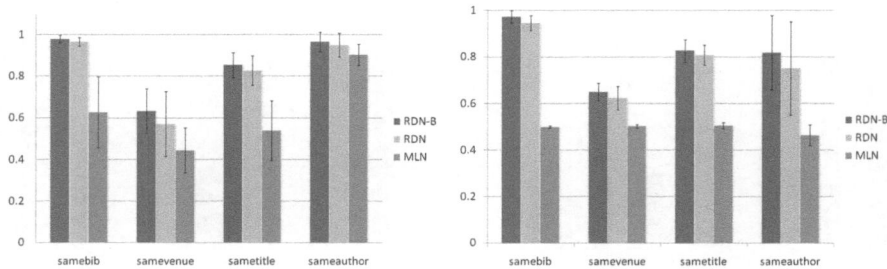

Fig. 3.4 Area under curves for the entity-resolution task in Cora dataset. The first graph shows the PR curve results while the second one is the area under curve for ROC curves

that was performed in the journal article (Natarajan et al 2012b). The paper contains expanded experimental section that compares relational regression trees vs relational probability trees, compares the use of boosting vs no boosting on several other data sets.

This chapter presented the first non-parameteric approach to relational density estimation: we turned the problem of learning RDNs into a series of relational function approximation problems using gradient-based boosting. We have shown that this non-parametric view on statistical relational learning allows one to efficiently and simultaneously learn both the structure and the parameters of RDNs. A keen reader might have observed that the intermediate structures are not always clearly interpretable. While this is true, we can always 'compile' the final structures it into 'single tree per predicate' models that are indeed comprehensible. Boosting has been previously explored in the context of propositional graphical models. Building on this success, we have outlined their adaptation to a relational probabilistic model. Next we show how to boost MLNs.

Chapter 4
Boosting Undirected Relational Models

Having presented the outline of functional gradient based learning of Relational Dependency Networks in the previous chapter, we turn our focus to learning undirected SRL models. More precisely, we adapt the algorithm for learning the popular formalism of Markov Logic Networks. We derive the gradients in this case and present empirical evidence to demonstrate the efficacy of this approach.

4.1 Introduction

Recall that Markov Logic Networks (MLNs) extend the undirected propositional representation of Markov networks to relational setting by expressing the knowledge as a set of weighted formulas. One of the nice features of MLNs is that they allow the user to write many rules about the domain and then learn weights for the rules to perform inference. In many cases, however, it is difficult to come up with all the rules. Subsequently, the task of learning the rules themselves (i.e., performing structure learning) is an important and challenging task and has received much attention lately (Biba et al. 2008; Mihalkova and Mooney 2007; Kok and Domingos 2009, 2010). As mentioned in Chap. 2, all these methods perform a two step process of first learning the structure (rules), then optimize the parameters (weights) and repeat until convergence.

Also recall that the process of functional gradient boosting is triggered by the intuition that finding many rough rules of thumb can be faster and more accurate than finding a single, highly accurate local model. Thus in the previous chapter, we turned the problem of learning relational models (more precisely RDNs) into a series of relational function approximation problems using functional gradient-based boosting. We represented each conditional probability distribution as a sum of regression models grown incrementally.

Following a similar approach, we learn a single MLN as a series of relational regression models. We use two kinds of representations for the functional gradients on the pseudo-likelihood for MLNs: *clauses* and *trees*. The former version simply learns a set of clauses at each gradient step each with an associated regression value

© The Author(s) 2014
S. Natarajan et al., *Boosted Statistical Relational Learners*,
SpringerBriefs in Computer Science, DOI 10.1007/978-3-319-13644-8_4

while the latter version views MLNs as a set of relational regression-trees. We present
both the methods and evaluate them on the standard SRL data sets.

We will demonstrate in this chapter the superior performance of boosting, both in
terms of time and accuracy of the learned model. Our approach also has the advantage
of learning more predictive rules than the many MLN structure learning algorithms.
In spite of learning more rules, our algorithms have smaller running times compared
to the state-of-the-art MLN algorithms. We believe that in several domains it is not
possible to obtain complete domain knowledge as a set of clauses and in such cases,
it is important to learn a better predictive model.

We now derive the gradients for the MLN and present the two different types
of regression models. We then present empirical evaluations before concluding the
chapter with a brief discussion.

4.2 Functional Gradients for MLNs

Recall that an MLN consists of a set of formulas in first-order logic and their real-
valued weights, $\{(w_i, f_i)\}$. The joint probability distribution over all atoms can now
be computed as

$$P(X = x) = \frac{1}{Z} \exp\left(\sum_i w_i n_i(x)\right) \tag{4.1}$$

where $n_i(x)$ is the number of times the ith formula is satisfied by possible world x
and Z is a normalization constant (as in Markov networks). Intuitively, a possible
world where formula f_i is true one more time than a different possible world is e^{w_i}
times as probable, all other things being equal.

Consider the joint probability equation, the conditional probability of an example,
say x_i given its Markov blanket ($\mathbf{MB}(x_i)$) can represented as:

$$P(x_i = true|\mathbf{MB}(x_i)) = \frac{\exp\left(\sum_j w_j n_j(x_i = true; MB(x_i))\right)}{\sum_{x'} \exp\left(\sum_j w_j n_j(x_i = x'; MB(x_i))\right)}$$

$$= \frac{\exp\left(\sum_j w_j nt_j(x_i; \mathbf{MB}(x_i))\right)}{\exp\left(\sum_j w_j nt_j(x_i; \mathbf{MB}(x_i))\right) + 1} \tag{4.2}$$

where we can define

$$nt_j(x_i; \mathbf{MB}(x_i)) \equiv n_j(x_i = true; \mathbf{MB}(x_i)) - n_j(x_i = false; \mathbf{MB}(x_i)) \tag{4.3}$$

$n_j(\mathbf{x})$ is the number of true groundings of clause C_j in the ground Markov network of
$\mathbf{x}$. Given our definition of the probability of an example, we can derive the potential

function ψ.

$$P(x_i|\mathbf{MB}(x_i)) = \frac{\exp\left(\psi(x_i;\mathbf{MB}(x_i))\right)}{\exp\left(\psi(x_i;\mathbf{MB}(x_i))\right)+1} = \frac{\exp\left(\sum_j w_j nt_j(x_i;\mathbf{MB}(x_i))\right)}{\exp\left(\sum_j w_j nt_j(x_i;\mathbf{MB}(x_i))\right)+1}$$

$$\Rightarrow \psi(x_i;\mathbf{MB}(x_i)) \equiv \sum_j w_j\, nt_j(x_i;\mathbf{MB}(x_i)) \tag{4.4}$$

In the above equation, $nt_j(x_i)$ is the difference between the number of true groundings of the clause C_j when an example is true and the groundings when it is false. If x_i appears in the head of a Horn clause C_j, $nt_j(x_i)$ also corresponds to the number of *non-trivial groundings* of x_i. Our prior work (Shavlik and Natarajan 2009) defined the notion of non-trivial groundings. Let us for example consider a clause say, $p(A,B) \wedge q(B,C) \rightarrow target(A)$. It can be easily observed that $target(c1)$ only appears in the head of the clause and hence $nt_j(target(c1))$ corresponds to the number of non-trivial groundings of $target(c1)$. Since this is a horn clause, it can be satisfied by either setting p or q to false. However, if either of these predicates are false, there is no effect on the final conditional distribution. Hence, the number of non-trivial groundings are the number of groundings of the *target* where the two other predicates are true.

As mentioned in the background chapter, most of the learning algorithms optimize the pseudo-log-likelihood (PLL) instead of the full log-likelihood.

$$PLL(\mathbf{X} = \mathbf{x}) = \sum_{x_i \in \mathbf{x}} \log P(x_i|\mathbf{MB}(x_i)) \tag{4.5}$$

Now, taking the derivative of PLL w.r.t. the function ψ, we get

$$\frac{\partial PLL(\mathbf{X} = \mathbf{x})}{\partial \psi(x_i = 1; \mathbf{MB}(\mathbf{x_i}))} = \frac{\partial \log P(x_i;\mathbf{MB}(\mathbf{x_i}))}{\partial \psi(x_i = 1; \mathbf{MB}(\mathbf{x_i}))}$$

$$= I(x_i = 1; \mathbf{MB}(\mathbf{x_i})) - P(x_i = 1; \mathbf{MB}(\mathbf{x_i}))\square \tag{4.6}$$

Note that the gradient at each example is now simply the adjustment required for the probabilities to match the observed value (x_i) for that example. This gradient serves as the weight for the current regression example at the next training episode. This is quite similar to the gradient step of the RDN case. Another way of understanding this concept at a fairly high-level is that the use of pseudolikelihood for MLNs yields an approximation that is similar in spirit to the approximation of directed SRL models by RDNs. Hence, our method can be understood as learning a set of RDNs to represent an MLN.

So what is the difference between functional gradient learning of RDNs and MLNs? We can clearly observe that RDNs do not use the number of groundings to compute the probability distributions (recall that they simply used existential quantifiers and/or aggregators in the inner nodes) from the different regression trees. MLN probability distribution on the other hand, depends on the number of groundings of the clause. Hence, all the examples that reach the same leaf may not have the same distribution due to each example potentially having different number of groundings of the clause corresponding to the path taken.

The next obvious question is: How do the number of groundings affect the relational regression learner? Then answer is that it depends on the underlying representation. We will discuss two different representations for these gradients.

Representation of Functional Gradients for MLNs

As with the case of RDNs, to apply functional gradient boosting, we need to find $\hat{\psi}$ such that the squared error between $\hat{\psi}$ and the functional gradient is minimized over all examples, i.e.,

$$\arg \min_{\hat{\psi}} \sum_{i=1}^{n} (\hat{\psi}(x_i; MB(x_i)) - \Delta(x_i))^2 \tag{4.7}$$

We consider two representations of $\hat{\psi}$s: *trees* and *clauses*. As we show next, these two representations are closely related even if there are crucial differences between them.

Tree Representation

For this case, we use a relational regression-tree learner to fit the gradients on each example. It is easy to see that in any weighted (i.e., regression) tree, each path from the root to a leaf can be seen as a clause and the weight at the leaf corresponds to the weight of the clause. As an example, let us consider adding the literal $q(X,Y)$ to the tree at a node N. Let the current clause formed by the path from the root to the node N be $p(X) \to target(X)$. So adding $q(X,Y)$ splits the current clause to two clauses,

$$C_1 : p(X) \wedge q(X,Y) \to target(X)$$

$$C_2 : p(X) \wedge \forall Y \neg q(X,Y) \to target(X)$$

For all the examples that reach node N (i.e., p(X)=true), let $\mathcal{I}$ be the set of examples that satisfy $q(X,Y)$ and $\mathcal{J}$ be the ones that do not. Let w_1 and w_2 be the regression values that would be assigned to C_1 and C_2 respectively. Let $n_{x,1}$ and $n_{x,2}$ be the number of non-trivial groundings for an example x with clauses C_1 and C_2. The regression value returned for an example now depends on whether it belongs to $\mathcal{I}$ or $\mathcal{J}$. The regression function for the examples reaching node N can be defined as

$$\hat{\psi}(x_i) = n_{x_i,1} \cdot w_1 \cdot I(x_i \in \mathcal{I}) + n_{x_i,2} \cdot w_2 \cdot I(x_i \in \mathcal{J}) \tag{4.8}$$

and the squared error (SE) is

$$SE = \sum_{x \in \mathcal{I}} \left[n_{x,1} \cdot w_1 - \Delta_x \right]^2 + \sum_{x \in \mathcal{J}} \left[n_{x,2} \cdot w_2 - \Delta_x \right]^2$$

Taking the derivative w.r.t. the weights, we can calculate the optimum value for the weights at the leaf for a given split.

$$\frac{\partial}{\partial w_1} SE = \sum_{x \in \mathcal{I}} 2 \left[n_{x,1} w_1 - \Delta_x \right] n_{x,1} + 0 = 0 \Rightarrow w_1 = \frac{\sum_{x \in \mathcal{I}} \Delta_x \cdot n_{x,1}}{\sum_{x \in \mathcal{I}} n_{x,1}^2} \tag{4.9}$$

Fig. 4.1 Sample tree for
target(X)

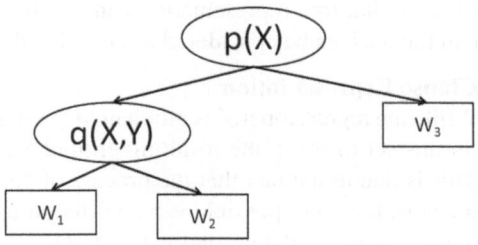

Since the optimum weights have a closed-form solution, we can compute the weights easily for possible literals that can be added at each node. We greedily search for the literal that minimizes the squared error with the optimum weights.

Figure 4.1 gives the sample regression tree for *target*(X) for the example considered above. Assume that the algorithm selected $p(X)$ to be the best split with weight w_3 on its false branch ($p(X) = false$) and it is scoring $q(X,Y)$ as the next split for the true branch. As described above, $\mathcal{I}$ contains all examples that have at least one grounding for $q(X,Y)$. $\mathcal{J}$ contains the rest of examples. *target*(x_1) is in $\mathcal{I}$ if $p(x_1) \wedge \exists Y q(x_1, Y)$ is true and *target*(x_2) is in $\mathcal{J}$, if $p(x_2) \wedge (\forall Y, \neg q(x_2, Y))$ is true. Given the number of groundings and gradients of examples in $\mathcal{I}$, we can now compute the weight w_1 on the left leaf using Eq. 4.9 and similarly compute w_2 on the right leaf by plugging in the number of groundings of $\mathcal{J}$ in the same equation.

Note that for the above relational regression tree, there is an equivalent MLN:

$$w_1 : p(X) \wedge q(X,Y) \rightarrow target(X)$$

$$w_2 : p(X) \wedge \forall Y \neg q(X,Y) \rightarrow target(X)$$

$$w_3 : \neg p(X) \rightarrow target(X) \tag{4.10}$$

Note that the examples reaching the leaf with weight w_1, namely $\mathcal{I}$, satisfy the body of the first clause. Also, by construction, these examples do not satisfy the body of the remaining two clauses. Recall that the non-trivial groundings of the clause correspond to the groundings which satisfy the body of the clause. Therefore, the set of examples $\mathcal{I}$ have zero non-trivial groundings for the last two clauses. Given our definition of ψ in Eq. 4.4, we can see that the weights of these clauses do not effect the regression value returned for examples in $\mathcal{I}$ (since $nt_j(x; \mathbf{MB}(x)) = 0$). Hence, we use the examples from $\mathcal{I}$ to only compute the weight for the first clause (where $nt_j(x; \mathbf{MB}(x)) > 0$). Similar to decision trees, we partition the examples into mutually exclusive sets and only use the examples reaching the leaf to efficiently calculate the weight at that leaf.

This is the key advantage of using a tree representation. Inherently, the tree representation becomes an ordered list of clauses as explained earlier. So when computing the probability of an example, we simply run through the list of clauses, find the first clause that it satisfies and use the weight and number of groundings for that clause in the probability calculation ignoring the rest of the clauses due to the definition of non-trivial groundings. For more details on the ordered list and the caveats in some cases, we refer to our journal paper. For the purposes of this book, it is sufficient to observe that tree representation can be quite efficient for MLNs and that the trees can themselves be considered as an ordered list of clauses.

Clause Representation

While the regression tree is efficient to learn, if we are to employ any MLN inference on this set of trees, the resulting ground Markov network can become quite large. This is due to the fact that the process of "grounding" creates a node in the ground network for every possible value of the grounding of the predicate. This can lead to a large clique in the ground network. Of course, this can be avoided if we perform lifted inference (Poole 2003; de Salvo Braz et al. 2005; Kersting et al. 2009; Singla and Domingos 2008; Kersting 2012) but that is out of the scope of this book.

To alleviate this problem, we define a second representation for the regression function, namely a set of Horn clauses. To learn this clausal representation, we ignore the false branch, i.e., set the weights on the false branch (w_2 and w_3 in the previous example) to zero. We learn Horn clauses by using a beam search that adds literals to clauses that reduce the squared error. We maintain a (beam-size limited) list of clauses ordered by their squared error and keep expanding clauses from the top of the list. We add literals to clauses as long as their lengths do not exceed a threshold and there are clauses in the stored list yet to be expanded. We recommend using the clausal representation when the existential variables introduced by the trees would make the inference step too slow.

In this version of boosting MLNs, we learn a set of clauses independently at each gradient step. Since we do not have two branches when every new condition is added, the error function becomes:

$$SE = \sum_{x \in \mathcal{I}} \left[n_{x,1} \cdot w - \Delta_x \right]^2 + \sum_{x \in \mathcal{J}} \Delta_x^2 \implies w = \frac{\sum_{x \in \mathcal{I}} \Delta_x \cdot n_{x,1}}{\sum_{x \in \mathcal{I}} n_{x,1}^2}$$

Note that the key change is that we do not split the nodes and instead just search for new literals to add to the current set of clauses. Hence, instead of an ordered-list of clauses, we learn a single clause obtained by taking the true branch at every node. We repeat this process to obtain a pre-set number of clauses (set to 3 in our experiments) within each gradient step.

Algorithm 2 FitRelRegressionTree(S, P):
Fit relational regression trees to the regression dataset, S.

```
 1: Tree := createTree(P(X))
 2: Beam := {root(Tree)}
 3: L := 8                                               ▷ Maximum leaves
 4: while numLeaves(Tree) ≤ L do
 5:     Node := popBack(Beam)                            ▷ Node with worst score
 6:     C := createChildren(Node)                        ▷ Create children
 7:     BN := popFront(Sort(C))                          ▷ Node with best score
 8:     addNode(Tree, Node, BN)                          ▷ Replace Node with BN
 9:     insert(Beam, BN.left, BN.left.score)
10:     insert(Beam, BN.right, BN.right.score)
11: end while
12: return Tree
```

Overall Algorithm for Boosting MLNs

Algorithm 2 presents the pseudocode for learning relational regression trees for MLNs. The function $FitRelRegressionTree(S, P)$ corresponds to the function used in Algorithm 7. We limit our trees to have maximum L leaves and greedily pick the worst node to expand (to reduce the error in that node). In $FitRelRegressionTree$, we begin with an empty tree that returns a constant value. We use the background predicate definitions to create the potential literals that can be added ($createChildren$). We pick the best scoring node (based on square error) and replace the current leaf node with the new node ($addNode$). Then both the left and right branch of the new node are added to the potential list of nodes to expand. To avoid overfitting, we only insert and hence expand nodes that have at least six examples. We pick the node with the worst score and repeat the process.

$FitRelRegressionClause(S, P)$ is called instead of $FitRelRegressionTree$ when learning clauses. $FitRelRegressionClause$ uses the maximum clause length as the parameter N (we set this to 3) and beam size B (we set this to 10). We greedily try to find the best scoring clause (BC) with $length \leq N$. In every iteration, we pick the current best performing clause from a queue for expansion. We add all the clauses that improve the score to our queue, while only keeping the best B clauses in the queue and ignoring the rest. We repeat this process till no expansions of clauses with $length \leq N$ are possible. Note that this method only learns one clause at a time. Hence for learning multiple clauses, we call this function multiple times during one gradient step and update the gradients before each call based on the currently learned clauses. In general, we learn a maximum of three clauses in a single gradient step.

Algorithm 3 FitRelRegressionClause(S, P):
Fit relational regression clauses to the dataset, S.

```
 1: Beam := {P(X)}                                          ▷ Initialize with the target predicate
 2: BestClause := P(X)
 3: N := 3                                                      ▷ Maximum clause length
 4: B:= 10                                                            ▷ Beam width
 5: while ¬empty(Beam) do
 6:     Clause := popFront(Beam)              ▷ Pick the best scoring clause to expand
 7:     if length(Clause) ≥ N then
 8:         continue                                      ▷ Clause too long to be expanded
 9:     end if
10:     C := addLiterals(Clause)              ▷ Possible expansions of the base clause
11:     for c ∈ C do
12:         c.score = SE(c)                          ▷ Score of the expanded clause c
13:         if c.score ≥ Clause.score then
14:             insert(Beam, c, c.score)      ▷ Add the expansion if it is better than the base clause
15:         end if
16:         if c.score ≥ BC.score then
17:             BestClause := c                          ▷ Update best scoring clause
18:         end if
19:     end for
20:     while [ doConsider the best B clauses to expand]length(Beam) ≥ B
21:         pop(Beam)
22:     end while
23: end whilereturn BC
```

4.2.1 Learning Joint Models

From the way we currently presented our learning algorithm, it would appear to the reader that we are learning clauses for a single target predicate. One of the key features of probabilistic models in general and SRL models in particular, is the ability to learn and reason about predicates and examples jointly.

To handle multiple target predicates in the case of MLNs, we learn a joint model by learning tree/clauses for each predicate in turn. We use the MLN clauses learned for all the predicates prior to the current iteration to calculate the regression value for the examples. For example while learning the joint model for three predicates p, q and r, we iterate through each predicate and learn one tree at a time. Lets assume we iterate through the predicates in the order $\{p, q, r\}$ and we have learned the kth tree for q. When computing the gradients for predicate r, we use the $k - 1$ trees learned for r along with the k trees learned for p and q. Also for efficiency, while learning a tree for the target predicate r, we do not consider the influence of that new tree on other target predicates p and q. While learning a model with a single target predicate, all the Horn clauses in that model have the target predicate as the head of the clause. We have shown the efficiency and correctness of this approach in a related paper (Khot et al. 2014).

4.3 Empirical Evaluation

We now present the evaluation on the three data sets that we have introduced. For more experiments and results, we refer to our related papers (Khot et al. 2011, 2014). We compared the two versions of our boosting algorithms—tree-based (MLN-BT) and clause-based (MLN-BC) to four state-of-the-art MLN structure learning methods: LHL (Kok and Domingos 2009), BUSL (Mihalkova and Mooney 2007), Motif-S (short rules) and Motif-L (long rules) (Kok and Domingos 2010). In addition, we also compared against a hand coded MLN for which we simply learned weights either using discriminative learning denotes as Alch-D or generative learning denoted as Alch-G.

We employed the default settings of Alchemy (Kok et al. 2010) for weight learning on all the datasets, unless mentioned otherwise. We set the $multipleDatabases$ flag to true for weight learning. For inference, we used MC-SAT sampling with 1 million sampling steps or 24 h whichever occurs earlier. For learning structure using motifs, we used the settings provided by Kok and Domingos (Kok and Domingos 2010). While employing LHL and BUSL for structure learning, we used the default settings in Alchemy. We set the maximum number of leaves in MLN-BT to 8 and maximum number of clauses to 3 in MLN-BC. The beam-width was set to 10 and maximum clause length was set to 3 for MLN-BC. We used 20 gradient steps on all the boosting approaches.

Table 4.1 Results on UW data set. Higher values are better

Algo	2X negatives		All negatives		Time
	AUC-PR	CLL	AUC-PR	CLL	
MLN-BT	**0.94 ± 0.06**	**−0.52 ± 0.45**	0.21 ± 0.17	−0.46 ± 0.36	18.4 s
MLN-BC	**0.95 ± 0.05**	**−0.30 ± 0.06**	0.22 ± 0.17	−0.47 ± 0.14	33.3 s
Motif-S	0.43 ± 0.03	−3.23 ± 0.78	0.01 ± 0.00	−0.06 ± 0.03	1.8 h
Motif-L	0.27 ± 0.06	−3.60 ± 0.56	0.01 ± 0.00	−0.07 ± 0.02	10.1 h
Alch-D	0.31 ± 0.10	−3.90 ± 0.41	0.01 ± 0.00	−0.08 ± 0.02	7.1 h
LHL	0.42 ± 0.10	−2.94 ± 0.31	0.01 ± 0.01	−0.06 ± 0.02	37.2 s

MLN-BT boosting with trees, *MLN-BC* boosting with clauses, *Motif-S* motif with short rules, *Motif-L* motif long rules, *Alch-D* hand-coded rules with discriminative learning, *LHL* lifted hypergraph learning

4.3.1   UW Data Set

For this data set, Table 4.1 presents the AUC and CLL values, along with the training time taken by each method averaged over 5-folds. The training time does not change for the different test-sets. As can be seen, for the complete dataset both boosting approaches (MLN-BT and MLN-BC) perform significantly better than other MLN learning techniques on the AUC-PR values. Current MLN learning algorithms on the other hand are able to achieve lower CLL values over the complete dataset by pushing the probabilities to 0, but are not able to differentiate between positive and negative examples as shown by the low AUC-PR values. We could not get BUSL to run on this data set.

When we reduce the negatives in the test set to twice the number of positives, the boosting techniques dominate on both the AUC-PR and CLL values, while the other techniques, which cannot differentiate between the examples, have poor CLL values. Also, there is no significant difference between learning the trees or the clauses in the case of boosting MLNs.

Further experiments revealed that the performance of the algorithm did not improve after adding 20 trees. Hence, in all the experiments, we set a maximum of 20 trees to be learned.

4.3.2   Cora Data Set

For Cora, we learn a joint model over SameBib, SameVenue, SameTitle and SameAuthor. Since this dataset is large, to speedup learning we sampled 25 % of the examples during every gradient step for MLN-BT. Similar to the UW dataset, we used a handcoded MLN ($B+N+C+T$) for Cora presented by Singla et al. (2006). We evaluated all the models jointly over the four target predicates given the evidence predicates. We used the queryEvidence flag for Alchemy weight learning and inference. As with the previous case, we could not get BUSL to run on this data set.

We performed 5-fold cross-validation and averaged the results over all the folds. The AUC-PR and CLL values are presented in Table 4.2. MLN-BT has a slightly lower performance compared to MLN-BC since we need longer rules to accurately cluster entities. The entity-resolution task requires rules such as `Title(B1,T1)`, `Title(B2,T2)`, `SameBib(B1,B2)` → `SameTitle(T1,T2)` which the greedy approach used in boosting may never find. Since any subset of the given rule would have little impact on the squared error, MLN-BT never learn such rules. MLN-BT scores two literals at a time for a given node and as a result learns short rules that only capture common words between the titles. MLN-BC on the other hand searches for clauses of length 3 and hence may learn longer rules. Nevertheless, both methods are significantly better than other MLN learning methods. While structural Motifs and LHL methods are comparable when predicting the `SameAuthor` relationship, our boosting-based methods are significantly better for all the other relationships.

4.3.3   IMDB Data Set

For this data set, as with other experiments, we performed 5-fold cross validation. We used the folds generated by Mihalkova and Mooney (2007) and averaged the results across all the folds. We perform inference over every predicate given all other predicates as evidence.

Table 4.3 shows the AUC values for the three predicates: `workedUnder`, `genre` and `gender`. The boosting approaches perform better on average, on both the AUC and CLL values, than the other methods. The BUSL method seems to exhibit the best performance of the prior structure-learning methods in this domain. Our boosting algorithms seem to be comparable or better than BUSL on all the predicates. For `workedUnder`, LHL has comparable AUC values to the boosting approaches, while it is clearly worse on the other predicates. There is no significant difference between the two versions of the boosting algorithms.

We also asked another interesting question in this domain: how do boosted MLNs compare against boosted RDNs (Natarajan et al. 2012b)? So, we compared our proposed methods against boosted RDNs (RDN-B). As can be seen from Table 4.3, the MLN-based methods are marginally better than the boosted RDNs for predicting `workedUnder` predicate, while comparable for others. This is a significant finding in that there is not much difference between learning of MLNs and RDNs in terms of performance. But RDN learning can be much more effective and simpler even though they are approximations.

Table 4.2 Results on the Cora testbed

Algorithm	AUC-PR				CLL			
	SameBib	SameVenue	SameTitle	SameAuthor	SameBib	SameVenue	SameTitle	SameAuthor
MLN-BT	**0.96 ± 0.02**	0.56 ± 0.17	0.71 ± 0.20	0.96 ± 0.04	−0.39 ± 0.04	−5.32 ± 1.88	−8.09 ± 2.97	−0.29 ± 0.14
MLN-BC	**0.96 ± 0.02**	0.68 ± 0.09	**0.82 ± 0.13**	0.98 ± 0.02	−0.33 ± 0.06	−5.12 ± 3.86	−11.18 ± 7.28	−0.60 ± 0.39
Alch-G	0.63 ± 0.17	0.45 ± 0.11	0.54 ± 0.14	0.90 ± 0.05	−5.58 ± 1.49	−4.27 ± 0.96	−5.14 ± 1.39	−8.87 ± 0.37
Alch-D	0.63 ± 0.17	0.48 ± 0.12	0.58 ± 0.16	0.92 ± 0.06	−4.95 ± 0.06	−4.08 ± 1.14	−4.34 ± 0.82	−3.32 ± 1.82
Motif-S	0.63 ± 0.16	0.45 ± 0.10	0.61 ± 0.17	0.93 ± 0.09	−2.54 ± 1.45	−1.80 ± 1.57	−2.79 ± 1.36	−1.57 ± 1.63
LHL	0.63 ± 0.17	0.45 ± 0.10	0.52 ± 0.15	0.91 ± 0.04	−5.99 ± 1.60	−4.20 ± 0.97	−5.11 ± 1.41	−8.80 ± 0.34

Table 4.3 Results on IMDB data set

	AUC-PR			CLL		
Algorithm	workedUnder	genre	gender	workedUnder	genre	gender
MLN-BT	0.90 ± 0.07	0.94 ± 0.08	0.45 ± 0.06	-0.18 ± 0.06	-0.20 ± 0.09	-0.62 ± 0.05
MLN-BC	1.00 ± 0.00	1.00 ± 0.00	0.39 ± 0.07	-0.11 ± 0.04	-0.12 ± 0.08	-0.84 ± 0.21
RDN-B	0.99 ± 0.02	0.91 ± 0.12	0.46 ± 0.18	-0.88 ± 0.20	-0.25 ± 0.22	-0.76 ± 0.16
BUSL	0.89 ± 0.11	0.94 ± 0.08	0.44 ± 0.08	-0.56 ± 0.05	-0.27 ± 0.09	-0.69 ± 0.01
LHL	1.00 ± 0.00	0.37 ± 0.09	0.39 ± 0.12	-0.02 ± 0.01	-1.13 ± 0.23	-0.73 ± 0.05
Motif-S	0.56 ± 0.16	0.52 ± 0.29	0.48 ± 0.08	-2.73 ± 1.66	-3.99 ± 2.70	-0.71 ± 0.08
Motif-L	0.48 ± 0.27	0.39 ± 0.03	0.46 ± 0.08	-2.30 ± 1.16	-2.32 ± 1.15	-0.69 ± 0.06

4.4 Discussion

Since MLNs provide clear semantics and convergent inference approaches (Singla and Domingos 2008), they are among the most popular SRL methods. But learning the rules of MLNs remains one of the hardest and challenging problems. We address the problem of structure learning by using gradient-boosting with the added benefit of learning weights simultaneously. A similar approach has been taken independently in the propositional world for learning Markov Networks by Lowd and Davis (2010). They learn Markov network structure as a series of local models where each local model is a set of decision trees. Our proposed approach can be seen as generalizing their approach to learning MLNs by using functional gradient boosting.

Building upon the success of pseudo-likelihood methods for MLNs, we derived tree-based and clause-based gradient boosting algorithms. We demonstrated on the three tasks the efficacy of the learning algorithm. The results yielded an interesting insight - the connection to RDN learning. As can be observed in the experiments, the performance is not too different from the results presented in the previous chapter. A natural question is then, which formulation is better? The answer is not straightforward. While at a high-level glance it might appear that RDNs may be the right model because of efficiency of existentials and aggregators, it is not always the case. Recall that our inference process for MLNs is cumbersome. This is due to the fact that we completely ground the entire network and perform propositional inference. As mentioned earlier, lifted inference methods can avoid many of the problems with this inference method. When combined with an approximate counting method, they can be quite efficient. In such cases, MLNs might be preferable as they are not approximate models like RDNs. Currently, both models are interesting and have their own benefits when applied to real data.

Chapter 5
Boosting in the Presence of Missing Data

The learning approaches presented in the last two chapters employed the closed-world assumption i.e., whatever that is not observed in the data is assumed to be false. In this chapter, we relax this assumption and derive a boosting algorithm that can effectively work with missing data. The derivation is independent of the model and hence we will discuss about adapting it for RDNs and MLNs. As with other chapters, we will conclude with empirical evaluation on the SRL data sets.

5.1 Introduction

Research with missing data in SRL has mainly focused on learning the parameters (Natarajan et al. 2008). In such cases, algorithms based on classical EM (Dempster et al. 1977) have been developed for several SRL models such as ones with combining rules (Natarajan et al. 2008; Jaeger 2007) and PRISM (Kameya and Sato 2000). Li and Zhou(2007) directly learn the structure of a PRM model from hidden data. They use maximum-likelihood trees to iteratively fill the missing values and update the structure and use dependency analysis to learn the final structure. Since they are learning a directed model, they have to perform the expensive check of ensuring acyclicity in the ground model. Kersting and Raiko (2005) learn the structure of logical HMMs in presence of missing data. Their approach, inspired by Friedman's structural EM approach for Bayesian networks (Friedman 1998) computes the sufficient statistics over the hidden states and does a greedy hill-climbing search over the clauses.

We significantly extend this approach—inspired by the success of structural EM on propositional graphical models (Friedman 1998) and the success of boosting in learning SRL models, we propose an EM algorithm for functional-gradient boosting (FGB). We derive and present the update equations of the E and M-steps of the algorithm. One of the key features of our algorithm is that we consider the set of distributions in the models to be a product of potentials and this allows us to learn different models such as MLNs (Domingos and Lowd 2009; Khot et al. 2011) and RDNs (Neville and Jensen 2007; Natarajan et al. 2012b). After deriving the EM

© The Author(s) 2014
S. Natarajan et al., *Boosted Statistical Relational Learners*,
SpringerBriefs in Computer Science, DOI 10.1007/978-3-319-13644-8_5

algorithm, we adopt the standard approach of approximating the full likelihood by the MAP states (i.e., hard EM). We show that this MAP approximation to the likelihood makes learning computationally tractable with minimal change in quality. As far as we are aware, this is the first work on combining EM with FGB for relational domains.

5.2   Structural EM for Relational Functional Gradients

Recall that the Expectation-Maximization (EM) algorithm for standard graphical models proceeds in two steps. In the first "E" step, the expected values of the missing attributes are computed based on the current structure and parameters. These expected values are used in "M" step where the parameters (and possibly structure) are determined that maximize the loglikelihood. In the next iteration, new expected values are computed and the new parameters (and possibly structure) are obtained. The process repeats till convergence. Given this background, we now present our version of EM algorithm that is combined with FGB.

Let us denote the observed data using $\mathbf{X}$ and the hidden data using $\mathbf{Y}$. Also, let us use 1 and 0 to represent true and false respectively. Given a training set with missing data, the goal is to maximize the log likelihood of the observed groundings. We average the likelihood function over all possible world states of the missing data (joint assignment over all hidden groundings) to compute the marginal probabilities of the observed groundings as shown below.

$$\ell(\psi) \equiv \log P(\mathbf{X} = \mathbf{x}|\psi) \qquad \rhd \text{ Likelihood } (\ell) \text{ of observed data } \mathbf{x}$$

$$= \log \sum_{\mathbf{y} \in \mathcal{Y}} P(\mathbf{x}; \mathbf{y}|\psi) \qquad \rhd \text{ Marginalize over hidden data instantiations}$$

$$= log \sum_{\mathbf{y} \in \mathcal{Y}} \left\{ P(\mathbf{y}|\mathbf{x}; \psi') \frac{P(\mathbf{x}; \mathbf{y}|\psi)}{P(\mathbf{y}|\mathbf{x}; \psi')} \right\} \qquad \rhd \text{ Multiply and divide by } P(\mathbf{y}|\mathbf{x}; \psi')$$

$$(5.1)$$

Assume ψ' is our current estimate of the best model based on the log-likelihood function. We will derive gradient steps to find ψ that has a higher log-likelihood than ψ'. We then set the ψ obtained via these gradient steps as the new ψ' and iteratively find a better ψ. To make the iterative procedure clearer, we use ψ_t to represent the ψ' obtained after t iterations of the gradient steps.

Before we provide further technical details of the algorithm, we present the high-level overview of our RFGB-EM (Relational Functional Gradient Boosting - EM) approach in Fig. 5.1. Similar to EM approaches that we explained earlier, we sample the states for the hidden groundings based on our current model in the E-step and use the sampled states to update our model in the M-step. ψ_t represents the model in the tth iteration. The initial model, ψ_0 can be as simple as a uniform probability for all examples or could be a model specified by an expert. We sample certain number of

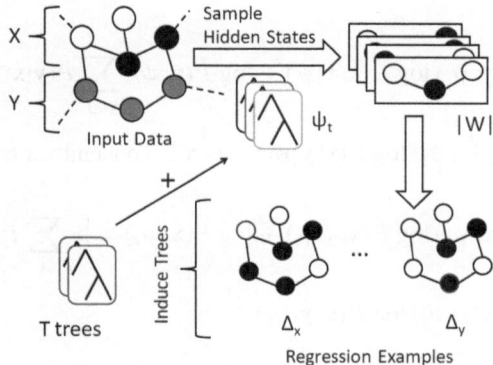

Fig. 5.1 RFGB-EM flowchart. *Shaded nodes* indicate variables with unknown assignments, while the *white* (or *black*) nodes are assigned true (or false) values. The input data has observed (indicated by **X**) and hidden (indicated by **Y**) groundings. We sample $|W|$ assignments of the hidden groundings using the current model ψ_t. We create regression examples based on these samples, which are used to learn T relational regression trees. The learned trees are added to the current model and the process is repeated

assignments of the hidden groundings (denoted as $|W|$) using the current model ψ_t. Based on these samples, we create regression examples which are then used to learn T relational regression trees. The learned regression trees are added to the current model and the process is repeated.

Similar to the RFGB approach presented in the previous chapters, we can start with a simple prior or some expert advice as the initial model, ψ_0. Unfortunately maximizing the log likelihood function directly is not feasible and so we maximize the lower bound on $\ell(\psi)$. To find the lower bound, we first rewrite Eq. 5.1 using ψ_t,

$$\ell(\psi) = log \sum_{\mathbf{y} \in \mathcal{Y}} \left\{ P(\mathbf{y}|\mathbf{x}; \psi_t) \frac{P(\mathbf{x}; \mathbf{y}|\psi)}{P(\mathbf{y}|\mathbf{x}; \psi_t)} \right\}$$

$$\geq \sum_{\mathbf{y} \in \mathcal{Y}} P(\mathbf{y}|\mathbf{x}; \psi_t) log \frac{P(\mathbf{x}; \mathbf{y}|\psi)}{P(\mathbf{y}|\mathbf{x}; \psi_t)} \qquad \triangleright \text{ Jensen's Inequality}$$

$$= \sum_{\mathbf{y} \in \mathcal{Y}} P(\mathbf{y}|\mathbf{x}; \psi_t) log \frac{P(\mathbf{x}; \mathbf{y}|\psi) P(\mathbf{x}|\psi_t)}{P(\mathbf{x}; \mathbf{y}|\psi_t)} \qquad \triangleright \text{ P(A} | \text{B)} = \text{P(A, B) / P(B)}$$

$$= \sum_{\mathbf{y} \in \mathcal{Y}} P(\mathbf{y}|\mathbf{x}; \psi_t) log P(\mathbf{x}; \mathbf{y}|\psi) + \sum_{\mathbf{y} \in \mathcal{Y}} P(\mathbf{y}|\mathbf{x}; \psi_t) log P(\mathbf{x}; \psi_t)$$

$$- \sum_{\mathbf{y} \in \mathcal{Y}} P(\mathbf{y}|\mathbf{x}; \psi_t) log P(\mathbf{x}; \mathbf{y}|\psi_t)$$

$$= \sum_{y \in \mathcal{Y}} P(\mathbf{y}|\mathbf{x}; \psi_t) \log P(\mathbf{x}; \mathbf{y}|\psi) + \log P(\mathbf{x}; \psi_t) \sum_{y \in \mathcal{Y}} P(\mathbf{y}|\mathbf{x}; \psi_t)$$

$$- \sum_{y \in \mathcal{Y}} P(\mathbf{y}|\mathbf{x}; \psi_t) \log P(\mathbf{x}; \mathbf{y}|\psi_t) \qquad \triangleright \mathbf{x} \text{ is constant w.r.t. } \mathbf{y}$$

$$= \sum_{y \in \mathcal{Y}} P(\mathbf{y}|\mathbf{x}; \psi_t) \log P(\mathbf{x}; \mathbf{y}|\psi) + \log P(\mathbf{x}; \psi_t) \qquad \triangleright \sum_{A} P(A \mid B) = 1$$

$$- \sum_{y \in \mathcal{Y}} P(\mathbf{y}|\mathbf{x}; \psi_t) \log P(\mathbf{x}; \mathbf{y}|\psi_t)$$

The second term matches the log-likelihood function that we started with, except it is defined for ψ_t instead of ψ. The first and third term have similar form except for variations in the model used (ψ or ψ_t). To simplify these terms, we define a function $\mathcal{Q}$ as

$$\mathcal{Q}(\psi) \equiv \sum_{y \in \mathcal{Y}} P(\mathbf{y}|\mathbf{x}; \psi_t) \log P(\mathbf{x}; \mathbf{y}|\psi) \qquad (5.2)$$

We can now rewrite the lower bound of $\ell(\psi)$, derived above, as

$$\ell(\psi) \geq \mathcal{Q}(\psi) + \ell(\psi_t) - \mathcal{Q}(\psi_t) \qquad (5.3)$$

Instead of finding ψ that maximizes $\ell(\psi)$, it is easier to find the ψ that maximizes this lower bound. Since ψ_t is constant with respect to the parameter ψ, we only need to find the ψ that maximizes $\mathcal{Q}(\psi)$. However, in many situations, finding a ψ that improves over $\mathcal{Q}(\psi_t)$ would suffice, since it will ensure that ψ has a higher log-likelihood than ψ_t as shown below.

$$\mathcal{Q}(\psi) \geq \mathcal{Q}(\psi_t)$$
$$\Rightarrow \mathcal{Q}(\psi) - \mathcal{Q}(\psi_t) \geq 0$$
$$\Rightarrow \mathcal{Q}(\psi) - \mathcal{Q}(\psi_t) + \ell(\psi_t) \geq \ell(\psi_t)$$
$$\Rightarrow \ell(\psi) \geq \ell(\psi_t) \qquad \triangleright \text{From Eq. 5.3}$$

Hence in our iterative procedure, the $\mathcal{Q}$ function value and consequently the log-likelihood increases or stays the same after every iteration. Since there is no closed-form solution for finding the ψ function that maximizes $\mathcal{Q}(\psi)$, we use steepest descent with functional gradients. Running steepest descent until convergence would find the maxima of the $\mathcal{Q}(\psi)$ function (which might be a local maxima for some functions). Note that a single step of gradient descent with functional gradients involves learning one tree for every predicate. Running functional-gradient descent until convergence would result in learning a large number of trees for just one update to ψ_t. Thus, instead of maximizing the $\mathcal{Q}(\psi)$ function, we take few gradient steps (two in practice) to find the ψ function. We then use this ψ function as the base model ψ_t for the next iteration.

To derive the functional gradients, consider the definition of $\mathcal{Q}$ function

$$\mathcal{Q}(\psi) \equiv \sum_{\mathbf{y} \in \mathcal{Y}} P(\mathbf{y}|\mathbf{x}; \psi_t) \log P(\mathbf{x}; \mathbf{y}|\psi)$$

The second term in this equation is the joint likelihood of the observed data and an assignment for the missing data. Recall from the previous two chapters that the joint distribution is considered as a product of conditionals for learning both RDNs and MLNs. If we denote the joint distribution as $P(\mathbf{z}; \psi)$. Then it is simply the product of conditionals $\prod_{z \in \mathbf{z}} P(z \mid \mathbf{z} \setminus z; \psi)$. We use Z as the union of all the variables i.e. $Z = X \cup Y$. As mentioned in the background chapter, we use $\mathbf{z}_{-z}$ to denote $\mathbf{z} \setminus z$ and $\mathcal{Y}_{-i}$ to represent the world states for the set of groundings $\mathbf{y}_{-y_i}$ (i.e. $\mathbf{y} \setminus y_i$). Hence we can now rewrite $\mathcal{Q}(\psi)$ as

$$\mathcal{Q}(\psi) = \sum_{\mathbf{y} \in \mathcal{Y}} P(\mathbf{y}|\mathbf{x}; \psi_t) \sum_{z \in \mathbf{x} \cup \mathbf{y}} \log P(z|\mathbf{z}_{-z}; \psi)$$

Once we have this expression, the next natural step is the computations of gradients for each example. Note that these gradients have to be computed for both the hidden and observed groundings of the hidden and target predicates. The value returned by the ψ function also depends on other ground literals, since their values will influence the path taken in the regression tree. In the previous chapter, we included them as arguments to the function definition, i.e. $\psi(x; \mathbf{MB}(x))$. But $\mathbf{MB}(x)$ is observed and has the same values across all examples (the blanket varies across examples but the ground literal's Boolean values are the same) and so the function can be simplified to $\psi(x)$. However, with missing data, the assignment to the hidden variables $\mathbf{y}$ is not constant because each assignment to $\mathbf{y}$ may return a different value for a given example (due to different paths taken by examples). Hence, we include the assignment to the hidden variables in our function ($\psi(x; \mathbf{y})$) and compute the gradients for an example and hidden-state assignment.

5.2.1   Gradients for Hidden Groundings

First we will derive the groundings of the hidden predicates before proceeding to deriving the gradients for the observed groundings. The gradients of $\mathcal{Q}$ w.r.t. the hidden groundings can be obtained by taking partial derivatives of $\mathcal{Q}$ w.r.t $\psi(y_i; \mathbf{y}_{-i})$, where y_i is a hidden grounding. The value of $\psi(y_i; \mathbf{y}_{-i})$ is only used to calculate $P(y_i|\mathbf{x}, \mathbf{y}_{-i}; \psi)$ for two world states: where y_i is true and where y_i is false. So the gradient w.r.t. $\psi(y_i; \mathbf{y}_{-i})$ can be calculated as

$$\frac{\partial \mathcal{Q}(\psi; \psi_t)}{\psi(y_i; \mathbf{y}_{-i})} = P(y_i = 1, \mathbf{y}_{-i}|\mathbf{x}; \psi_t) \frac{\partial \log P(y_i = 1|\mathbf{x}, \mathbf{y}_{-i}; \psi)}{\partial \psi(y_i; \mathbf{y}_{-i})}$$

$$+ P(y_i = 0, \mathbf{y}_{-i}|\mathbf{x}; \psi_t) \frac{\partial \log P(y_i = 0|\mathbf{x}, \mathbf{y}_{-i}; \psi)}{\partial \psi(y_i; \mathbf{y}_{-i})}$$

As shown before, the gradients would correspond to the difference between the true value of y_i and the current predicted probability of y_i (i.e. $I(y_i = y) - P(y_i = y)$). As we have terms involving $P(y_i)$ for each value of y_i, we get two gradient terms.

$$P(y_i = 1, \mathbf{y}_{-i} | \mathbf{x}; \psi_t)(1 - P(y_i = 1 | \mathbf{x}, \mathbf{y}_{-i}; \psi))$$
$$+ P(y_i = 0, \mathbf{y}_{-i} | \mathbf{x}; \psi_t)(0 - P(y_i = 1 | \mathbf{x}, \mathbf{y}_{-i}; \psi))$$
$$= P(y_i = 1, \mathbf{y}_{-i} | \mathbf{x}; \psi_t) - P(\mathbf{y}_{-i} | \mathbf{x}; \psi_t) P(y_i = 1 | \mathbf{x}, \mathbf{y}_{-i}; \psi)) \tag{5.4}$$

With the PLL assumption, the gradients can be written as $\prod_{j \neq i} P(y_j | \mathbf{x}, \mathbf{y}_{-j}; \psi_t)$ $\left[P(y_i = 1 | \mathbf{x}, \mathbf{y}_{-i}; \psi_t) - P(y_i = 1 | \mathbf{x}, \mathbf{y}_{-i}; \psi) \right]$. Intuitively, the gradients correspond to the difference between the probability predictions weighted by the probability of the hidden-state assignment.

5.2.2   Gradients for Observed Groundings

To compute the gradients for the observed groundings, we take partial derivatives of Q with respect to $\psi(x_i; \mathbf{y})$, where x_i is observed in the data. Similar to the gradients for hidden groundings, we use $\mathbf{y}$ as an argument in the ψ function and only consider the world states that match with the given argument. The gradient w.r.t. $\psi(x_i; \mathbf{y})$ is calculated as

$$\frac{\partial Q(\psi; \psi_t)}{\psi(x_i; \mathbf{y})} = P(\mathbf{y} | \mathbf{x}; \psi_t) \frac{\partial \log P(x_i | \mathbf{x}_{-i}, \mathbf{y}; \psi)}{\partial \psi(x_i; \mathbf{y})}$$
$$= P(\mathbf{y} | \mathbf{x}; \psi_t)[I(x_i) - P(x_i = 1 | \mathbf{z}_{-x_i}; \psi)] \tag{5.5}$$

Similar to the hidden groundings, the gradients correspond to the difference between the predictions weighted by the probability of the hidden-state assignment.

5.2.3   Algorithm for Boosting in Presence of Hidden Data

We now present the basic pseudo-code for our RFGB-EM (Relational Functional Gradient Boosting - EM) approach in Algorithm 4. The function, ψ_t represents the model in the tth iteration. We perform T iterations of the EM algorithm, where we fix $T = 10$ since results did not change much after 10 iterations in our experiments.

Algorithm 4 RFGB-EM:
Expectation-Maximization algorithm for RFGB to handle missing data.

Require: Hidden literals, H
Require: Observed literals, D
 1: Set initial model, ψ_0
 2: t := 0
 3: **for** $t < T$ **do**
 4:     W := sampleWorld(H, D, ψ_t)   ▷ E-step
 5:     ψ_{t+1} := updateModel(W, D, ψ_t)   ▷ M-Step
 6: **end for**
 7: return ψ_T

We present the algorithm for updating the model in Algorithm 5. In the E-step we simply sample the values for hidden groundings. The *updateModel* (W, D, ψ) function corresponds to the M-step. As mentioned before, we do not run gradient descent till convergence in our M-step. Typically, we take $S = 2$ gradient steps to find a better scoring model rather than the best possible model. This allowed us to amortize the cost of sampling the world states and run enough EM iterations in reasonable time without making the model too large.

Algorithm 5 updateModel(W, D, ψ):
Update the model ψ based on sampled states, W.

1: $S := 2$ ▷ Number of trees learned in M-step
2: **for** $i \leq S$ **do**
3:     **for** [**do**Iterate over target and hidden predicates, P]$_p \in P$
4:         $E_p := sampleExamples(D, p)$ ▷ Downsampled groundings of p
5:         $D_p := buildDataset(E_p, W, D, \psi)$
6:         $T_p := learnTree(D_p, D)$
7:         $\psi = \psi + T_p$
8:     **end for**
9: **end for**
10: return ψ

Since each gradient step learns one tree, we learn $S \times T$ trees for each predicate after T EM iterations, which would be 20 trees in our case. We cycle over all the query and hidden predicates and learn one tree for each predicate per gradient step. We compute the gradients for the groundings of predicate p given by E_p, using the

---

Algorithm 6 buildDataset(E_p, W, D, ψ):
Build regression dataset for boosting.

1: $D_p := \emptyset$
2: **for** [**do**Iterate through examples]$e \in E_p$
3:     $\Delta_e := 0$
4:     **for** [**do**Iterate through sampled worlds]$w \in W$
5:         $\Delta_e := gradient(e, w)$
6:         $D_p := D_p \cup < e, \Delta_e >$
7:     **end for**
8: **end for**
9: return D_p

---

world states W, observed data D and current model ψ. We then learn a relational regression tree using this data set and add it to our current model.

The input examples to our regression tree learner are of the form $< (z; \mathbf{y}), \Delta >$. For every ground literal $z \in \mathbf{x} \cup \mathbf{y}$, we calculate the gradients for an assignment to the hidden variables. Algorithm 6 describes the *buildDataset* function used to compute the gradients for the examples. For every ground literal e and every world state w

(i.e., **y**), we compute the gradient of the example $(gradient(e, w))$. For examples that are observed, we use Eq. 5.5 to compute $gradient(e, w)$ and for examples that are hidden, we use Eq. 5.4.

Computing probabilities for all possible world states would be exponential in the number of hidden groundings. This would also result in computing the gradients for all examples for each one of these world states. Hence we use Gibbs sampling to generate $|W|$ samples from the distribution $P(\mathbf{y}|\mathbf{x}; \psi_t)$ to approximate all the world states, $\mathcal{Y}$. Since our gradients are weighted by the probability of the hidden-state assignment, an unlikely assignment will result in small gradients and thereby have little influence on the learned tree. Hence, we can sample the most likely hidden-state assignments to approximate the gradients. This is analogous to the Monte Carlo Expectation Maximization (MCEM) approach used for high dimensional data (Wei and Tanner 1990). We refer to this approximation of the RFGB-EM approach as SEM-W (S stands for *Structural*), where W is the number of worlds sampled. SEM-1 corresponds to sampling the most likely assignment and corresponds to the hard-EM approach.

Note that adapting the proposed EM algorithm to the cases of learning RDNs and MLNs is relatively straightforward. RDNs approximate the joint as product of conditionals while for MLNs we use the PLL approximation for the full likelihood. The only difference is in the counts and the inference tasks. So the adaptation is straightforward to these settings. For details, we refer to our journal paper (Khot et al. 2014).

5.3 Empirical Evaluation

We now present our empirical evaluation on two data sets—UW-CSE and IMDB. In these two domains, we learn the structure of RDNs. The two versions SEM-10 (ten sampled worlds) and SEM-1 (hard-EM) are compared against the standard method of applying closed-world assumption (i.e., use the method presented in Chap. 3 and simply consider whatever is unobserved as false). We present only RDN learning for coherence. For details on MLN learning experiments and experiments with other settings, we refer to our paper (Khot et al. 2014).

5.3.1 UW Data Set

For this data set, we randomly hid groundings of the `tempAdvisedby`, `inPhase`, and `hasPosition` predicates during training. Due to these hidden groundings and the different type of SRL model being learned, our numbers are not exactly comparable to the ones reported in previous chapters. We performed five-fold cross-validation and present the CLL values in Table 5.1. We do not present the AUC PR values since the difference is not statistically significant. We also varied the amount

Table 5.1 CLL values for UW-CSE

Hidden %	20 %	40 %
SEM-10	**−0.168**	**−0.170**
SEM-1	**−0.150**	**−0.151**
CWA	−0.187	−0.192

Table 5.2 CLL values for IMDB

Hidden %	10 %	20 %
SEM-10	**−0.501**	**−0.551**
SEM-1	**−0.423**	**−0.467**
CWA	−0.586	−0.80

of hidden data in our experiments ("Hidden %" in the table indicates the percentage of the groundings being hidden).

In general, the EM methods perform statistically significantly (with p-value <0.05) better than the closed-world assumption. It appears that in this domain, using a single sample for the hidden state has the same performance as that of using ten samples. This is in line with most EM algorithms, where using a single state (MAP) approximation generally suffices.

5.3.2 IMDB Data Set

For this data set, we predicted the gender predicate given all the other predicates. We randomly hid the groundings of actor and workedUnder predicates during learning and inference. Again due to these hidden predicates, our numbers are not comparable to the ones reported earlier. We performed 5-fold cross-validation.

We present the CLL values for hiding 10 % and 20 % of the groundings of the two hidden predicates in Table 5.2. Similar to the disjunctive dataset, there is no statistically significant difference between any two of the three methods in the AUC-PR values and hence are not reported here. In general, the EM methods perform statistically significantly (with p-value < 0.05) better than the closed-world assumption. Between the two EM methods, using one sample is sufficient to capture the underlying distribution and, hence, SEM-1 has a higher CLL value than SEM-10.

5.4 Discussion

We addressed the challenging problem of learning SRL models in the presence of hidden data. We developed an EM-based algorithm for functional-gradient boosting. We derived the gradients for the M-step by maximizing the lower bound of the gradient and showed how to approximate the E-step. Due to the fact that we approximate the joint as a product of conditional distributions, several different models can be adapted in this formulation. Our results indicate that the proposed algorithms outperform the respective algorithms that make closed-world assumptions.

We end this chapter on a more sober note. While theoretically interesting, we had a few interesting observations about the practical nature of this algorithm. An astute reader must have noticed that we did not present the evaluations on the Cora data set. This is due to two reasons: the first is that learning can be very expensive requiring significantly large computation time. But the second reason is more important and pertinent. In this domain, the relations are quite sparse. Which means that most of the relations are false. Hence, treating most of the hidden groundings as false already yields a very good model. This implies that the closed world assumption is sufficiently accurate in this task (as with several relational tasks).

To understand this better, consider an unary relation (relation with one argument). If there are n values, then this relation can take n groundings. Treating some of the missing ones as being false can have an adverse effect. But as the arity of the relations grows, the number of true groundings of the relation can become relatively small compared to the total number of groundings. For instance a ternary relation such as with 100 grounding per argument, can have the total possible groundings as 10^6. The total number of true groundings on the other hand is significantly smaller than a million groundings. And thus treating most of them as false is not unreasonable compared to the unary relation. Our experiments have confirmed that the proposed approach is robust when the arity is small and the network is dense. For longer relations and sparse networks, original RFGB algorithm with closed-world assumption is equally accurate.

Chapter 6
Boosting Statistical Relational Learning in Action

In the previous chapters, we discussed the structure learning algorithms for two SRL models and extended them to learn with missing data. In this chapter, we discuss how this algorithm can be adapted to learn to act in sequential domains. We then present three of our most successful applications in real health care data—two cardiovascular prediction problems and the third is prediction of onset of Alzheimer's disease. We then conclude the chapter with a few NLP applications.

6.1 Adaptation to Sequential Decision Making Problems

Kersting and Driessens (2008) addressed the problem of learning policies (selecting actions) in relational domains and posed this learning problem using functional-gradient boosting. To this effect, they considered a specific type of solution technique called as policy-gradient that compute the gradient of expected reward with respect to the parameters of the policy. In essence, they directly manipulate the policy instead of an implicit representation such as value function. The key idea in this work is to employ the boosting approach to represent the policy as a sum of relational-regression trees. Specifically, their algorithm samples a few episodes starting from the current state and regresses on the policy learned in the previous gradient step. A new tree is induced in the current gradient step. Experimental results in relational domains show significant improvement over current policy gradient methods. The learning procedure employed in this book for the different SRL models is inspired from this prior work.

6.1.1 Relational Imitation Learning

We addressed the problem of imitation learning in relational domains (Natarajan et al. 2011). Imitation learning refers to the problem of learning how to behave by observing a teacher in action and has been typically formulated as learning a

© The Author(s) 2014
S. Natarajan et al., *Boosted Statistical Relational Learners*,
SpringerBriefs in Computer Science, DOI 10.1007/978-3-319-13644-8_6

representation of a policy—a mapping from states to actions—from examples of that policy. Most sequential decision making problems are formulated as Markov Decision Processes (MDPs).

An MDP is described by a set of discrete states $\mathbf{S}$, a set of actions $\mathbf{A}$, a reward function $r_s(a)$ that describes the expected immediate reward of action a in state s, and a state transition function $p_{ss'}^a$ that describes the transition probability from state s to state s' under action a. A policy, π, is defined as a mapping from states to actions, and specifies what action to execute in each state. In the learning from demonstrations setting (i.e., imitation learning), we assume that the reward function is not directly obtained from the environment. Our input consists of S, A and supervised trajectories is generated by a Markov policy, and we try to match it using a parameterized policy. We assume a predicate logic notation for states and actions (parameterized). Hence, the input is a set of $\langle state, action \rangle$ trajectories. The goal is to induce a policy $P(a|s)$ that best mimics the expert.

We assume a set of training instances $\{\langle \mathbf{f_i^j}, a_i \rangle_{i=1}^{m^j} \}_{j=1}^{n}$ that is provided by the expert. Given these training instances, the goal is to learn a policy μ that is a mapping from $\mathbf{f_i^j}$ to a_i^j for each set of features $\mathbf{f_i^j}$. Since we are in the relational setting (we consider domains such as blocksworld, a real-time strategy game, traffic control with multiple agents and the breakaway sub-task of Robocup soccer), the individual features are considered to be relational. The features are denoted in standard logic notation where $p(X)$ denotes the predicate p whose argument is X.

It should be reasonably clear by now that the learning problem can be formulated as that of relational functional-gradient boosting. We consider learning a set of distributions for each parameterized action. For instance, if the actions are *moveUp(S)*, *moveDown(S)*, *moveLeft(S)* and *moveRight(S)* for each square say S in a grid world, we learn a set of trees for each of these predicates. So over all we learn 80 trees (20 trees per predicate). These trees will include the features of the state and essentially specify the probability of choosing each action given any set of state features. These different probabilities are then normalized to obtain a distribution over all the actions.

Our algorithm for imitation learning using functional gradient boosting is called as *TBRIL* and is presented in Algorithm 7. Note that this is very similar to boosting RDNs, except that instead of going through each predicate in turn, we go through each parameterized action in turn and boost its conditional distribution.

Algorithm *TBoost* is the main algorithm that iterates over all actions. For each action (k), it generates the examples for our regression tree learner (called using function *FitRRT*) to get the new regression tree and updates its model (Λ_m^k). This is repeated up to a pre-set number of iterations M (typically, $M = 20$). We found empirically that increasing M has no effect on the performance as the example weights nearly become 0 and the regression values in the leaves are close to 0 as well. Note that the after m steps, the current model Λ_m^k will have m regression trees each of which approximates the corresponding gradient for the action k. These regression trees serve as the individual components $(\Delta_m(k))$ of the final potential function. A key point about our regression trees is that they are not large trees. Generally, in our

---

Algorithm 7 TBRIL

```
 1: function TBOOST(Trajectories T)
 2:     for 1 ≤ k ≤ |A| do                                          ▷ Iterate through each action
 3:         for 1 ≤ m ≤ M do                                        ▷ M gradient steps
 4:             S_k := GenExamples(k; T; Λ^k_{m-1})
 5:             Δ_m(k) := FitRRT(S_k; L)                            ▷ Gradient
 6:             Λ^k_m := Λ^k_{m-1} + Δ_m(k)                         ▷ Update models
 7:         end for
 8:         P(A = k|f) ∝ ψ^k
 9:     end for
10: return
11: end function
12: function GENEXAMPLES(k, T, Λ)
13:     S := ∅
14:     for 1 ≤ j ≤ |T| do                                          ▷ Trajectories
15:         for 1 ≤ i ≤ |S^j| do                                    ▷ States of trajectory
16:             Compute P(â^j_i = k|f^j_i)        ▷ Probability of user action being the current action
17:             Δ_m(k; f^j_i) = I(â^j_i = k) − P(â^j_i = k|f^j_i)
18:             S := S ∪ [(â^j_i, f^j_i), Δ(â^j_i; f^j_i))]           ▷ Update relational regression examples
19:         end for
20:     end for
21: return S                                                        ▷ Return regression examples
22: end function
```

---

experiments, we limit the depth of the trees to be three and the number of leaves in each tree is restricted to be about eight (the parameter L in *FitRRT*). The initial potential Λ^1_0 is usually set to capture the uniform distribution in all our experiments. The function *GenExamples* (line 4) is the function that generates the examples for the regression-tree learner. As can be seen, it takes as input the current predicate index (k), the data, and the current model (Λ). It iterates over all the examples and for each example, computes the gradient based on the observed user action.

We performed experiments in several domains. We present only one of them for brevity. For more experiments, we refer to our prior work (Natarajan et al. 2011). The aim of Robocup soccer domain (Fig. 6.1a) (Stone and Sutton 2001) is to create a soccer team of robots that compete with each other. The state space is continuous and there is inherent uncertainty in the effects of actions. An action could, therefore, take the agent to one of a large number of next states. This is again a good domain for imitation learning because it is hard to explain what a good policy should look like but it is relatively easier to obtain expert data. Simplified versions of this game are run through a simulator which we use in this work.

For our experiments we collected data generated through the simulation of an expert policy for the M-on-N BreakAway (Torrey et al. 2007) where M attackers try to score a goal against N defenders. The attacker who has the ball may choose to move (ahead, away, left, or right with respect to the goal center), pass to a teammate, or shoot (at the left, right, or center part of the goal). RoboCup tasks are inherently multi-agent games, but a standard simplification is to have only one learning agent. This agent controls the attacker currently in possession of the ball, switching its focus

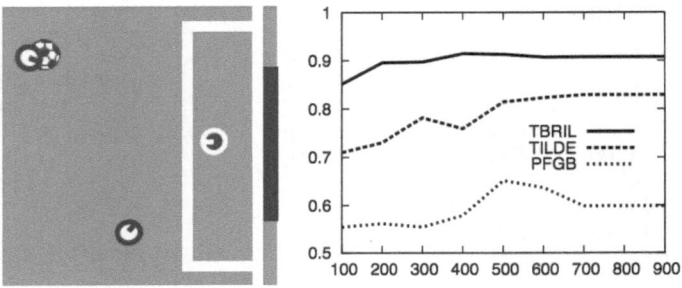

Fig. 6.1 a Robocup Domain. **b** AUC-PR vs. number of trajectories

between attackers as the ball is passed. Attackers without the ball follow simple hand-coded policies that position them to receive passes. The state information specifies the distances and angles between players and the goal post. We used the policies learned from an RL agent from the algorithm presented in (Torrey et al. 2007) as trajectories after the learner's policy has stabilized. This is particularly a challenging domain for RL since it involves mainly continuous features such as *distance* and *angle* between objects (players, ball and goal) and *time* which can lead to a large state space. We discretized these features to be used in the relational learner.

Figure 6.1b shows a comparison between the learning curves generated by *TBRIL*, *TILDE* tree learner and *propositional FGB* (PFGB). The area under the PR curve is averaged over the area for each of the seven actions. Yet again, the plot shows the superiority of *TBRIL*. The results in this problem shows that, as the problem complexity and hardness increase, so does the difference between the methods. *TILDE* and *PFGB* converges to a sub-optimal policy for the user while TBIRL has a very high precision and recall (close to 1) indicating that it can effectively mimic the user.

The key difference between this work and the work of Kersting and Driessens (2008) is that while the latter work requires the expensive step of using rewards to estimate policies and in turn estimate the value functions, in imitation learning, we can simply ignore the reward functions and instead focus on directly boosting the policies from trajectories.

6.2   Predicting Cardiovascular Events

The Coronary Artery Risk Developments in Young Adults (CARDIA) study is a longitudinal study of cardiovascular risk factors that began in 1985–1986. Participants have had comprehensive cardiovascular disease risk factors measured longitudinal with major exams every few years (1985, 1987, 1990, 1992, 1995, 2000, 2005, 2010) respectively. The purpose of this study is to understand the relationship between the measured risk factors and the development of advance cardio-vascular diseases. In particular, our prior work (Natarajan et al. 2013b) uses the longitudinal data collected from the CARDIA participants in early adult life, ages 20–50 years, to develop machine learning models that can be used to predict the Coronary Artery Calcification (CAC) amounts, an important indicator of cardiovascular disease, at years 25 given the measurements from the previous years.

We used known risk factors such as *age, sex, cholesterol, bmi, glucose, hdl level and ldl level of cholestrol, exercise, trig level, systolic bp and diastolic bp* that are measured between years 0 and 20 over the patients. Our goal is to predict if the CAC-levels of the patients are above 0 for year 20 given the above mentioned factors over all the years. Predicting the CAC-levels for year 20 using the measurements from previous years allows us to identify sub-groups of populations that are to be monitored early and identified for treatment and counseling. Any CAC-level over 0 indicates the presence of advanced coronary atheroma and elevated risk for future heart disease. So, we are in a binary classification setting of predicting 0 vs. non-0 CAC levels. In our data set, most of the population had CAC-level of 0 (less than 20 % of subjects had significant CAC-levels) in year 20. Hence there is a huge skew in the data set where there is a very small number of positive examples.

We used data from 3600 subjects and performed 5-fold cross validation. We compare the results (area under the curve of the ROC curves) of the SRL methods (presented below) against traditional regression methods linear and logistic regression. We boosted the conditional distribution of *P(CAC at year 20—all the measurements)* using RFGB. We also compare against standard machine learning methods such as Naive Bayes (John and Langley 1995), Support Vector Machines (Cristianini and Shawe-Taylor 2000), Decision trees (Quinlan 1993) (J48), a propositional boosting method (AdaBoost) (Freund and Schapire 1996) and relational probability trees (Neville et al. 2003a).

This is essentially a "rediscovery experiment" i.e., use known risk factors for predicting CAC levels. Preliminary results on CAC prediction task are presented in Fig. 6.2. As can be easily observed, the relational methods (RPT and RFGB) have a superior performance over the rest of the methods. In particular, the gradient boosting method (RFGB) exhibits more than 20 % increase over the best standard method. Our results are consistent with the published results (Craven and Shavlik 1996; Freund and Schapire 1996; Quinlan 1996) in that with about 25 trees, we can achieve the best empirical performance.

Figure 6.3 presents a part of one tree learned. We are not presenting the entire tree and indicate the missing branches by dots. The first argument a of every predicate is the subject's ID and the last argument of every predicate (except *sex*) indicates the year of measurement. The left branch out of every node is the *true* branch, the right branch the *false* branch. The leaves indicate the probability of CAC-level (say p) being greater than 0. We use *_bw* in predicates to indicate that the value of a certain variable is between two values. For instance, $ldl\_bw(a, b, 0, 100, 10)$ indicates that the LDL level of the person a is b and is between 0 and 100 in year 10. The leaves indicate the probability (p) of that subject having a non-zero CAC level in year 20. For example, the left branch states that if a person is male, he is in middle age in year 7 (i.e., between 35 and 45 years) and has a high ldl level, $p = 0.79$. Similarly the right branch indicates that if the subject is a female and has not smoked in year 5, $p = 0.05$.

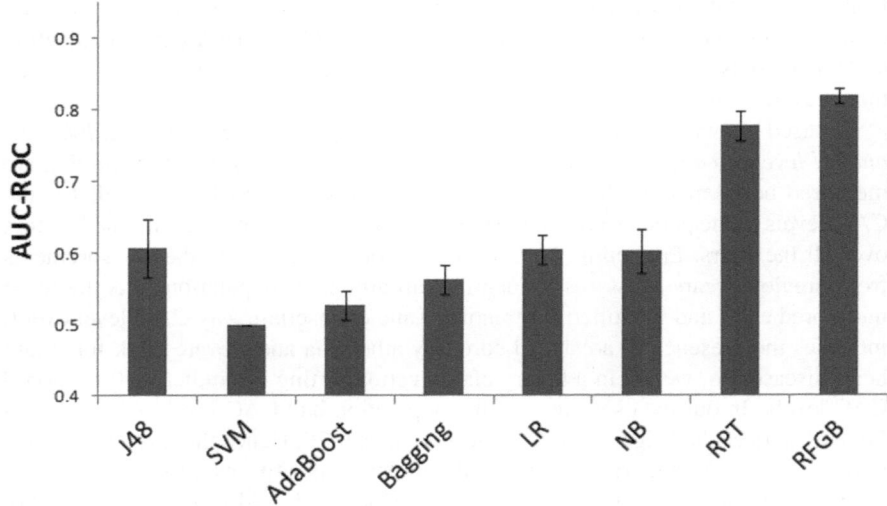

Fig. 6.2 AUC ROC values for the different algorithms

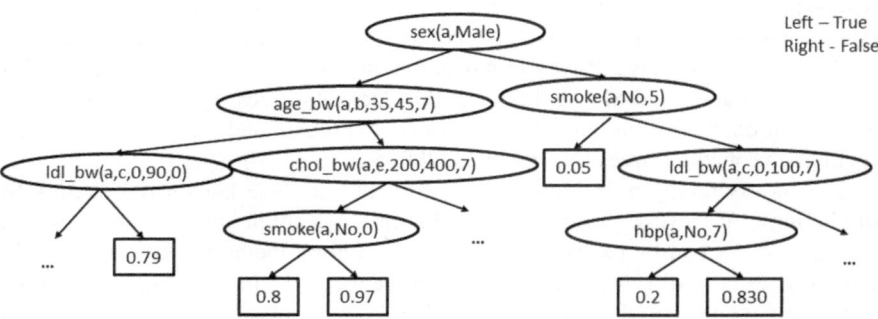

Fig. 6.3 Learned Tree for predicting CAC-level greater than 0. The leaves indicates $P(cac(a)) > 0$. The *left* branch at any test corresponds to test returning *true* while the *right* branch corresponds to *false*

We performed an additional experiment—we first used only year 0 data and learned a single tree. Now using this tree, we learned the second tree using year 5 data and so on. So the goal is to see how AUC-PR changes with adding more observations in future yeas and can be seen as the progress of the risk factor over time. The results are presented in Fig. 6.4 (solid). As expected from the previous experiment, year 0 has a big leap and then adding individual years increases performance till year 7 and then plateaus beyond that. This is again a significant result. Our initial results show that *beyond ages 25–37 of a person, there is not much significant information from the risk factors*. We refer to our work (Natarajan et al. 2013b) for

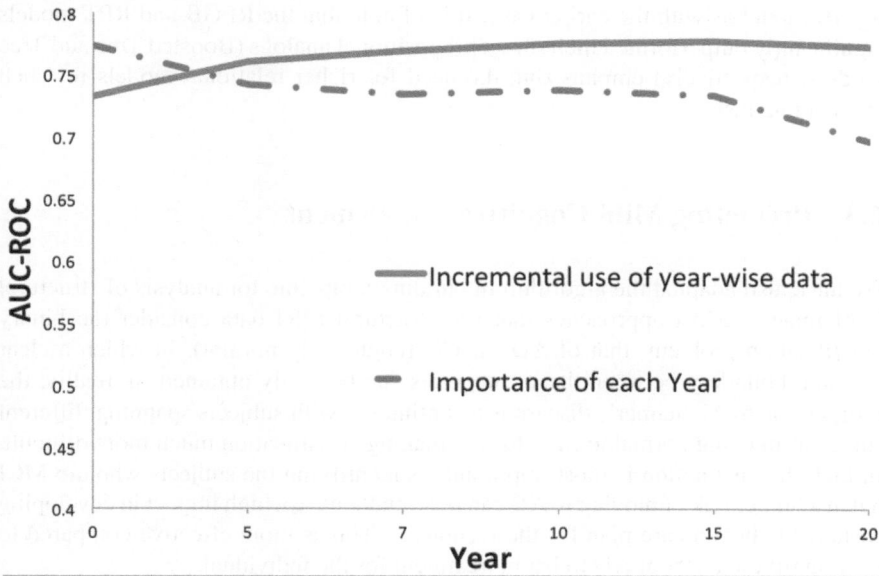

Fig. 6.4 The impact of the measurements in different years in the CAC-level at year 20

more details on the experiments, additional experiments and some perspectives on future research.

6.2.1   Application to a Real EHR

We have made an initial attempt of evaluating our algorithm on a real EHR (Weiss et al. 2012a, b). EHRs are an emerging data source of great potential use in disease prevention. An EHR effectively tracks the health trajectories of its patients through time for cohorts with stable populations. We analyzed de-identified EHR data on 18, 386 subjects enrolled in the Personalized Medicine Research Project (PMRP) at Marshfield Clinic (McCarty et al. 2005, 2008). The PMRP cohort is one of the largest population-based bio-banks in the United States and consists of individuals who are 18 years of age or older, who have consented to the study and provided DNA, plasma and serum samples along with access to their health information in the EHR. Most of the subjects in this cohort received most, if not all, of their medical care through the Marshfield Clinic integrated health care system. We included major risk factors such as cholesterol levels (LDL in particular), gender, smoking status, and systolic blood pressure, as well as less common risk factors such as history of alcoholism and procedures for echocardiograms and valve replacements. The best cross-validated predictor of primary MI according to AUC-ROC was the

RFGB model as with the earlier case. It is of note that the RFGB and RPT models significantly outperformed their direct propositional analogs (Boosted Tree and Tree models, respectively) emphasizing the need for richer relational models for such challenging tasks.

6.3   Predicting Mild Cognitive Impairment

We have also adapted the algorithm in building a pipeline for analysis of structural MRI images. Most approaches that use structural MRI data consider the binary classification problem, that of AD vs. CN (cognitively normal), in which a clear decision boundary between these categories can be easily obtained. In reality, the progression to Alzheimer's disease is a continuum, with subjects spanning different stages from being normal to MCI to AD, making classification much more difficult. In fact, this distinction is most important, as identifying the subjects who are MCI but at a higher risk of moving to AD can potentially have a high impact in developing sustainable health care plan for these subjects. This is more effective compared to waiting till the onset of AD to begin treatment for the individual.

Our approach (Natarajan et al. 2012a, 2013a) to addressing this problem involved a pipeline approach that performs three-way classification—AD vs. MC vs. CN. The pipeline is presented in Fig. 6.5 and consists of three stages—first is the *MRI segmentation stage* that takes MRI data as an input and segments the brain into clinically relevant regions. Second is a *relational learning stage* (RFGB) that considers the segmented brain to be a graph to build a series of binary classifiers. The final stage is the *combination stage* that combines the different classifiers. The idea underlying this pipeline is simple and is based on the idea of classical mixture of experts: rather than choose a single segmentation technique, we combine multiple segmentation techniques and different imaging data. We used an atlas based segmentation (AAL) which divides the brain into 116 regions.

We evaluate the pipeline on Alzheimer's Disease Neuroimaging Initiative (ADNI) database of 397 subjects. It should be mentioned that we did not carefully choose

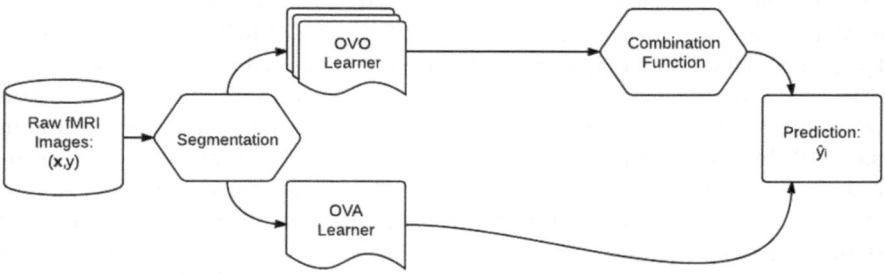

Fig. 6.5 Graphical representation of the pipeline for structural MRI analysis

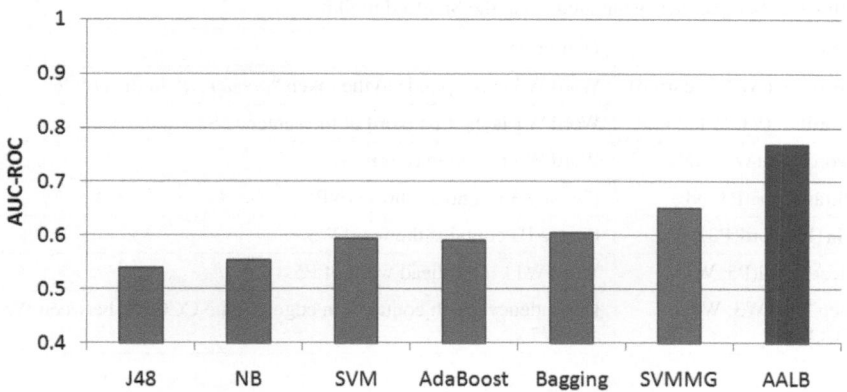

Fig. 6.6 Classification performances in terms of "Area under the ROC curve" of the different algorithms: propositional classifiers (*blue*) compared against the relational AALB (*red*) algorithm

the subjects for the study. This particular group was selected based upon having both structural MRI and functional metabolic positron emission tomography data as part of a separate study. Similarly, we do not perform careful feature selection but rather simply use resulting average tissue-type volume measurements obtained from the segmentation algorithms as features.

We now present the results in Fig. 6.6. All these classifiers used AAL segmentation to construct a feature vector and then performed classification using one of the standard machine learning methods (J48 - decision tree, NB - Naive Bayes, SVM - Support Vector Machine, AdaBoost and Bagging - ensemble classifiers). We used Weka and used the multi-class classification setting. For each of the classifiers, we used 5-fold CV to pick the best parameters. As can be seen, the propositional algorithms do not show a good performance when compared to AALB which is the SRL method (RFGB) used on top of the AAL segmentation method. We also present the results of running LibSVM on the voxel data (i.e., without any segmentation - SVMMG). As can be seen, the performance is slightly better but still is not comparable to the performance of AALB. As with the previous case study, we present AUC-ROC instead of accuracy.

6.4 NLP Applications

Finally, we briefly discuss three NLP applications where we have use our boosting approach.

Table 6.1 Sample facts generated using the Stanford toolkit

Example	Definition
WordText(W3, occurred)	Word W3 corresponds to the token *occurred* in the article
WordLoc(S1, W1, 1)	Word W1 is the first word of the sentence S1
WordType(W5, NN)	Word W5 is a noun (NN)
PhraseType(P3, NP)	Phrase P3 is a noun phrase (NP)
PhrHasWord(P3, W5)	Phrase P3 contains the word W5
HeadWord(P5, W11)	Word W11 is the head word of P5
DepType(W3, W7, CCOMP)	Dependency graph contains an edge of type CCOMP between W3 and W7

6.4.1 NFL Relation Extraction

We evaluate our method on another relation extraction task using the National Foot-ball League (NFL) dataset from the Linguistic Data Consortium[1] (LDC). This dataset consists of articles of NFL games over the past two decades. The idea is to read the texts and identify relations such as *score*, *team* and *game* in the text. For example, consider the text, "Green Bay defeated Dallas 28-14 in Saturday's Superbowl game." The goal is to identify *Green Bay Packers* and *Dallas Cowboys* as the teams, and 28 and 14 as their respective scores and the game to be a *Superbowl* game.

We generate *word-level*, *sentence-level*, *paragraph-level* and *article-level* rela-tional features from the Stanford NLP toolkit[2]. For each sentence, the Stanford NLP toolkit returns the tokenization, parse tree, dependency graph and named entity in-formation. We create a word object for each token in the sentence and a phrase object for each phrase in the parse tree. We create sentence- and paragraph-level features describing the number of words and position in the article. We also create article-level features such as the date of publishing and headline of the article. Table 6.1 presents a subset of the generated facts. Dependency paths[3] are considered to be important features for relation extraction and hence we create a special predicate to store the dependency path between every pair of words. Since there can be many such paths, we create the dependency path facts only if the path length is smaller than seven.

The area under curve for precision-recall ($AUCPR$) curves for the different rela-tions is presented in Fig. 6.7. As can be seen, for all the concepts, our boosted RDN method outperforms standard RDN learning method. As can be seen from the figure, while the concept of *score* is easier to learn, there is a lot of room for improvement for identifying the teams and the game. The key reason is that the natural text is quite ambiguous. For example, one article might mention the team as "San Francisco,"

---

[1] http://www.ldc.upenn.edu.

[2] http://nlp.stanford.edu/software/index.shtml.

[3] Dependency paths are paths in the dependency graph between a pair of entities.

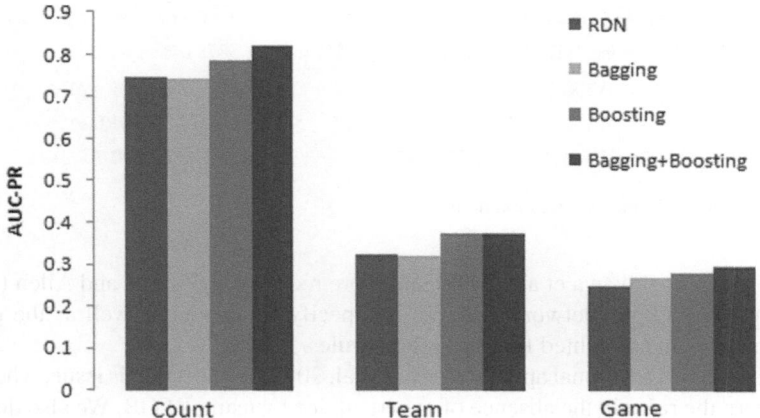

Fig. 6.7 Precision-Recall values for the NFL corpora. The results are presented for RDNs with a single RRT, Bagged RDNs, Boosted RDNs and Bagged, Boosted RDNs

the other article might mention them as "49ers" and the third article might use "SF 49ers." Hence, there is a need to perform co-reference resolution across articles.

6.4.2   Temporal Relation Extraction

Information extraction (IE) has been an important problem in the Natural Language Processing (NLP) community. One specific challenging IE problem is extraction of temporal ordering between events and temporal expressions. For example, for the sentence "He met the ambassador on June 3rd.", we would like to extract the relations OVERLAP ("met" , "June 3rd")and BEFORE ("met" ,DOCTIME), where DOCTIME corresponds to the document's creation time.

The TempEval dataset (Verhagen et al. 2007) uses six coarse-grained, temporal-ordering relations between events and timexes; between events and document creation time; and between events. Most of the approaches applied to the TempEval tasks use propositional features and independently learn relations for each task. However, learning to predict each task independently can lead to inconsistencies in the final prediction. For example, predicting event A happening before time T (A < T) and event B happening after time T (T < B) is inconsistent with event A happening after event B (A > B).

There have been approaches to handle these global inconsistencies during inference in propositional models (Chambers and Jurafsky 2008). By using SRL models, the relationships between the tasks and examples can also be specified using weighted rules to perform joint inference and thereby, ensure consistent ordering. These rules can even be included as part of the relational model before the learning step, rather than deferring the consideration of interaction among predictions to the inference

In [September]^{t239} , it [announced]^{e133} [plans]^{e134} to [acquire]^{e135} the tropical-fruit business
of RJR Nabisco Inc. 's Del Monte foods unit for #557 million ($878 million) .

Task C: e134 OVERLAP t239	Task E: e133 BEFORE e136
Task C: e133 OVERLAP t239	Task F: e134 BEFORE e135
Task C: e135 OVERLAP-OR-AFTER t239	Task F: e133 OVERLAP e134

Fig. 6.8 Sample TempEval-2 annotations

step. Hence, Yoshikawa et al. (2009) and more recently UzZaman and Allen (2010)
used Markov Logic Networks (MLNs) to specify the model as well as the global
constraints using weighted first-order logic rules.

We employ a relational approach (Khot et al. 2012) to address this issue, where we
also learn the rules in the absence of expert advice by using RFGB. We also develop
two extensions to leverage expert advice whenever available. Preliminary results of
our approach show promise for structure learning approaches in IE and other NLP
tasks.

6.4.2.1   TempEval tasks

Our work focused on the task of identifying relations between events and temporal expressions within the same sentence (called task C in TempEval-2). Figure 6.8
shows a sample TempEval-2 annotation, where tokens e133, e134 and e135 are
the event words whereas t239 marks a timex. In this example, since the announce-
ment happened in September, the annotations marked an OVERLAP relation between
e133 and t239.

We first use the Stanford NLP toolkit[4] to convert the documents into first-order
logic facts as presented before. We also convert the event and timex properties to
relational facts such as eventHasProperty(Event, Property, Value).
We then use these raw features to create richer features based on our analysis of the
domain. If provided, we also use expert advice such as the rules written by previous
work in this domain as the initial model. Given the initial model and the set of facts,
we use RFGB to learn a joint model for the target relations. Figure 6.9 presents our
approach.

6.4.2.2   Structure Learning for TempEval-2

Given the raw NLP features extracted from text, we use two forms of domain knowledge: (1) Specialized Features. We noticed that for most of the valid event-timex pairs
(i.e. having some relation), the event word is present in the dependency path (DP)

---

[4] http://nlp.stanford.edu/software/corenlp.shtml.

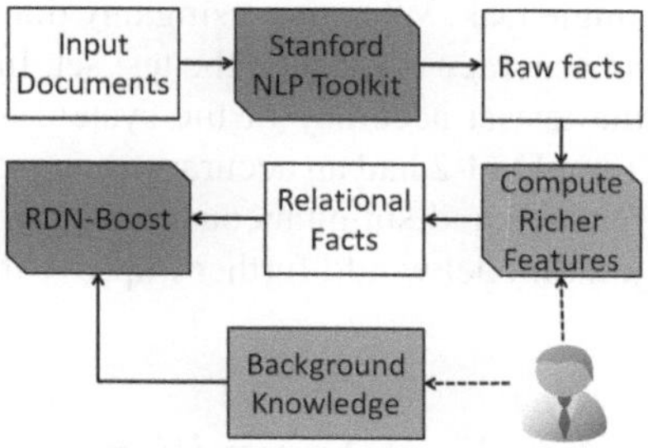

Fig. 6.9 Flowchart describing our approach for relation-extraction

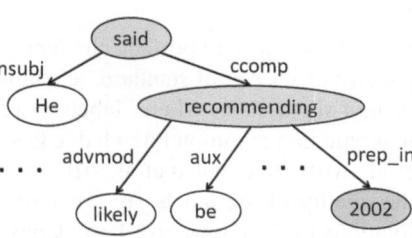

Fig. 6.10 Dependency graph for a sentence where OVERLAP relation exists between "*said*" and "*2002*"

from the timex to the root of the dependency graph (DG). Hence, if the DP goes up the tree and then goes down i.e. if there is a ↗↘ in the DP, then it is a strong signal that the event and timex are *not* related. We added a predicate `veeInDepPath(W1,W2)` which is true if neither W1 nor W2 is the ancestor of the other word. For example, in Fig. 6.10 we would create the fact: `veeInDepPath("be", " 2002")`.

Typically, a timex t is related to the first verb that appears in the DP from t to the root of the DG. However, additional verbs in the path to the root can also be related to t if they are preceded by special dependency tags (e.g. CCOMP). In order to learn such tags, we include a predicate `verbAlongDependencyPath` to represent this feature. We now let RDN-Boost discover which dependency types could be present for valid relations. Figure 6.10 shows a snippet of a DG. Although there is a verb in the DP from "2002" to "said," since "recommending" is connected by a CCOMP dependency type, "2002" applies to "said" too.

(2) Expert Rules. For the TempEval task, Yoshikawa et al. (2009) designed rules to encode the constraints for consistent ordering between events, timexes and document times. We use these rules as the initial model for RFGB. For example, consider the rule—relE2T(e1, t, "BEFORE") ∧ relE2T(e2, t, "AFTER") → relE2E(e1, e2, "BE-FORE"). This rule is used as the initial model for predicting relE2E. Here, relE2T represents relations between events and timexes and relE2E represents relations between events.

6.4.2.3 Preliminary Results

We present the preliminary results of our approach on task C of TempEval-2. We did not use any cross-task rules in the initial model, since we learn a model for a single task. When not using any domain-specific features, RFGB is able to achieve an accuracy of *0.56* on the test set. Including the domain-specific features improved the testset accuracy of the system to *0.60*. Most of the systems that competed in TempEval-2 had an accuracy ranging between 0.62 and 0.65. We believe with better features and simultaneously using the data from all the TempEval tasks to learn a joint model would further improve the results.

6.4.3 *Weak Supervision*

One of the most important challenges facing many natural language tasks is the paucity of the "gold standard" examples. An attractive and successful approach is *distant supervision* where, labels of relations in the text are created by applying a heuristic in a common knowledge base such as Freebase (Mintz et al. 2009; Riedel et al. 2010; Takamatsu et al. 2012). An important property of such methods is that the quality of the labels are crucially dependent on the heuristic used to map the relations to the knowledge base. Consequently, there have been several approaches that aim to improve the quality of these labels ranging from casting the problem as multi-instance learning (Riedel et al. 2010; Hoffmann et al. 2011) to using patterns that frequently appear in the text (Takamatsu et al. 2012).

We take a different approach of creating more examples to the supervised learner based on *weak supervision* (Craven and Kumlien 1999). We use commonsense knowledge to create sets of entities that are "potential" relations. This commonsense knowledge is written by a domain expert using MLNs. We then learns the parameters of these MLN clauses (we call them *world MLN*—WMLN—to reflect that they are non-linguistic models) from a knowledge base such as Wikipedia. During the information extraction phase, unlabeled text are then parsed through some entity resolution parser to identify potential entities. Then these entities are provided as queries to the world MLN which uses data from non-NLP sources such as Wikipedia to then predict the posterior probability of relations between these entities. These predicted relations become the probabilistic (weakly supervised) examples for RFGB.

While our approach has been presented in the context of information extraction, the idea of using outside world knowledge to create examples is more broadly applicable. For instance, this type advice can be used for labeling tasks (Torrey et al. 2010) or to shape rewards in reinforcement learning (Devlin et al. 2011) or to improve the number of examples in a medical task. Such advice can also be used to provide guidance to a learner in unforseen situations (Kuhlmann et al. 2004).

Our method consists of two distinct phases: *weak supervision phase* where we create weakly supervised examples based on commonsense knowledge and *information extraction phase* where we learn the structure and parameters of the models that predict relations using textual features.

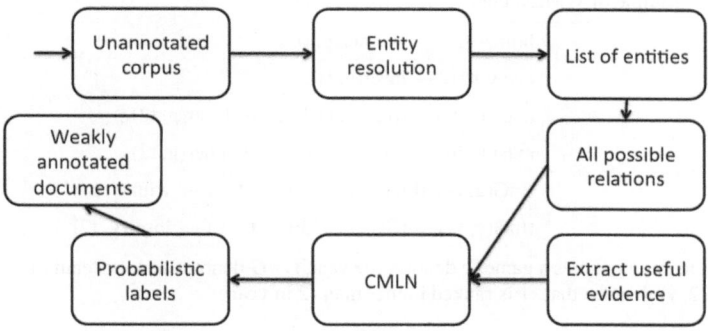

Fig. 6.11 Steps involved in creation of weakly supervised examples

6.4.3.1 Weak Supervision Phase

As mentioned earlier, the key challenge in information extraction is obtaining annotated examples. To address this problem, we employ a method that is commonly taken by humans. For instance, consider reading a newspaper sports section about a particular sport (say NFL). Before we even read the article, we have an inherent *inductive bias*—we expect a high ranked team (particularly if it plays at home) to win. In other words, we rarely expect "upsets". We aim to formalize this notion by employing a model that captures this inductive bias to label examples in addition to the gold standard examples. We use Markov Logic Networks (MLNs) to capture this world knowledge.

Our proposed approach for weak supervision is presented in Fig. 6.11. Our first step is to employ a MLN that captures some commonsense knowledge about the domain of interest, called as *WMLN*. For the NFL domain discussed earlier, some of the rules that we used are shown in Table 6.2. As can be observed from the table, our method uses some common knowledge such as "Home team is more likely to win the game" (first two clauses) and "High ranked team is more likely to win the game" (last two rules). Another clause that we found to be particularly useful is to say that "A team that is higher ranked and is the home team is more likely to win the game".

We learn the weights of these rules by extracting the previously played NFL games. Note that the rules are written without having the knowledge base in mind. These rules are simply written by the domain expert and they are softened using a knowledge base such as Wikipedia. The resulting weights are presented in the left column of the table. We used the games played in the last 20 years to compute these weights.

Note that one could simply define a higher ranking using the following MLN clause where t denotes a team, r its rank, y the year of the ranking and hR the higher rank: $\infty \quad rank(t1, r1, y), rank(t2, r2, y), t1! = t2, r1 < r2 \rightarrow hR(t1, t2, y)$.

Once the WMLN weights are learned, we proceed to create weakly supervised learning examples. We use the *Stanford NLP* toolkit to perform entity resolution to identify the potential teams, games and the year in sport articles. Once these entities

Table 6.2 A sample of WMLN clauses used for NFL task

0.33	home(g, t) → winner(g, t)
0.33	away(g, t) → loser(g, t)
∞	exist t2 winner(g, t1), t1 != t2 → loser(g, t2)
∞	exist t2 loser(g, t1), t1 != t2 → winner(g, t2)
0.27	tInG(g, t1), tInG(g, t2), hR(t1, t2, y) → winner(g, t1)
0.27	tInG(g, t1), tInG(g, t2), hR(t1, t2, y) → loser(g, t2)

t denotes a team, g denotes a game, y denotes the year, $tInG$ denotes that the team t plays in game g, $hR(t1, t2, y)$ denotes that $t1$ is ranked higher than $t2$ in year y

are identified, we query the WMLN for obtaining the posterior on the relations between these entities—for example, game winner and loser relations from NFL articles. We use the games that have been potentially played between the two teams (again from previously played games that year) to identify the home, away and ranking of the teams. We used the rankings at the start of the year of the game as a pseudo reflection of the relative rankings between the teams.

The result of the inference process are the posterior probabilities of the relations between the entities extracted in the documents. The resulting relations are then used as annotations. One simple annotation scheme is using the MAP estimate (i.e., if the probability of a team being a winner is greater than the probability of being the loser, the relation becomes positive example for winner and a negative example for loser). An alternative method would be to use a method that directly learns from probabilistic labels which we focus in this work by modifying the learning algorithm. Choosing the MAP would make a strong commitment about several examples on the borderline. Note that since our world knowledge is independent of the text, it may be the case that in some examples perfect labeling is not possible. In such cases, using a softer labeling method would be more beneficial. Now the examples are ready for our next step—learning the model for *information extraction.*

6.4.3.2 Learning for Information Extraction

Once the weakly supervised examples are created, the next step is inducing the relations. In order to do so, we employ the procedure presented in Fig. 6.12. We run both the gold standard and weakly supervised annotated documents through Stanford NLP toolkit to create relational linguistic features as mentioned earlier. Once these features are created, we run RFGB to learn a joint model between the target relations, for example, game winner and losers.

Since we use a probabilistic model to generate the weakly supervised examples, our training input examples will have probabilities associated with them based on the predictions from WMLN. We extend RFGB to handle probabilistic examples by defining the loss function as the KL-divergence between the observed probabilities

Fig. 6.12 Steps involved in learning using probabilistic examples

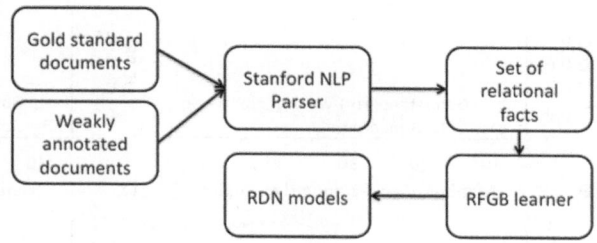

(shown using P_D) and predicted probabilities (shown using P). The functional gradients for the KL-divergence loss function can be shown to be the difference between the observed and predicted probabilities.

$$\Delta_m(x) = \frac{\partial}{\partial \psi_{m-1}} \sum_{\hat{y}} P_D(y = \hat{y}) \log \left(\frac{P_D(y = \hat{y})}{P(y = \hat{y} | \psi_{m-1})} \right)$$

$$= P_D(y = 1) - P(y = 1 | \psi_{m-1})$$

Hence we use probabilistic examples obtained from the weakly supervised phase as input to our structure learning phase along with gold standard examples (with $p = 1$ for positive examples), and their associated documents. Then a RDN is induced by learning to predict the different target relations jointly, using linguistic features created by the Stanford NLP toolkit.

6.4.3.3 Experimental Results

In this section, we present the results of our approach on the NFL domain. We compared the use of augmenting with weakly supervised examples against simply using the gold standard examples. Since we are also learning the structure of the model, we do not compare to other distant supervision methods directly but instead point out the state-of-the-art results in the problem.

Relation Extraction

In our evaluation, we consider only NFL articles that have annotations of positive examples. There were 66 annotations of the relations. We used 16 of these annotations as the test set and performed training on (a subset) rest of the documents. In addition to the gold standard examples, we used articles from the NFL website[5] for weak supervision. In our experiment, we wanted to evaluate the impact of the weakly supervised examples. We used 400 weakly supervised examples. We varied the number of gold standard examples while keeping the number of weakly supervised examples constant. In another setting, we used no weakly supervised examples and

---

[5] http://www.nfl.com.

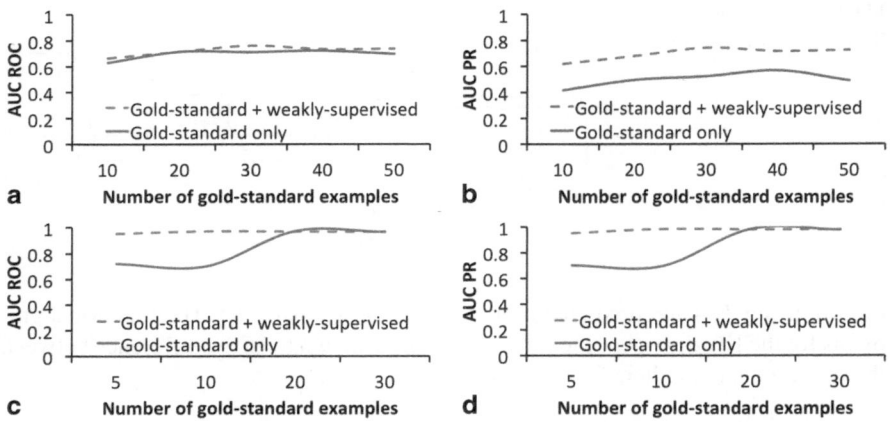

Fig. 6.13 Results of predicting winners and losers. **a** AUC ROC. **b** AUC PR. Document classification. **c** AUC ROC. **d** AUC PR

simply varied the number of gold standard examples. The results were averaged over five runs of random selection of gold standard examples.

We measured the area under curves for both ROC and PR curves. The results are presented in Fig. 6.13 where the performance measure is presented by varying the number of gold standard examples. As can be seen, in both metrics, the weakly supervised examples improve upon the usage of gold standard examples. The use of weakly supervised examples allows a jump start, a steeper learning curve and in the case of PR, a better convergence. It should be mentioned that while plotting every point, the set of the gold standard examples is kept constant for every run and the only difference is whether there are any weakly supervised examples added. For example, when plotting the results of 10 examples, for every run, the set of gold standard examples is the same. For the blue dashed curve, we add 400 more weakly supervised examples and this is repeated for runs in which the 10 gold examples are drawn randomly. We also performed t-tests on all the points of the PR and ROC curves. For the PR curves, the use of weakly supervised learning yields statistically superior performance over the gold standard examples for all the points on the curves (with p-value < 0.05). For the ROC curves, significance occurs when using 10, and 30 examples. Since PR curves are more conservative than ROC curves, it is clear that the use of these weakly supervised examples improves the performance of the structure learner significantly. To understand whether weak supervision clearly helps, we performed another experiment using a baseline where we randomly assigned labels to the 400 examples. When combined with 50 gold standard examples, the performance decreased dramatically with AUC values of 0.58 for both ROC and PR curves which clearly shows that the weakly supervised labels help when learning the structure.

Document Classification

To understand the general applicability of the proposed framework, we created another data set for evaluation. In this data set, the goal is to classify documents either as being *football(American)* or *soccer* articles. Hence the relation in this case is on the article (i.e.,*gametype(article,type)*). In order to do this, we extracted 30 football articles from the NFL website[6] and 30 soccer articles from the English Premier League (EPL) website[7] and annotated them manually as being football and soccer respectively. We used only the first paragraph of the articles for learning the models since it appeared that enough information is present in the first paragraph for learning an useful model. In addition, we used 45 articles for weak supervision. We used rules such as, "NFL teams play football", "EPL teams play soccer", "If the scores of both teams are greater than 10, then it is a football game", "If the scores of both teams are 0, then it is a soccer game".

All the rules mentioned above are essentially considered as "soft" rules. The weights of these rules were simply set to 100, 10, 1 to reflect the log-odds. Note that we could learn these weights as in the NFL cases, but the rules in this task are relatively simple and hence we simply set the weights manually. During the weak supervision phase, we used the entities mentioned in the documents as queries to the world MLN to predict the type of game that the entities correspond to. These predictions (probabilities) become the weak supervision for the learning phase. We labeled the 45 articles accordingly and combined them with the manually annotated articles.

As with the NFL data, we measured the AUC ROC and PR values by varying the number of gold standard examples. Again, in each run, to maintain consistency, we held the gold standard examples to be constant and simply added the weakly supervised examples. The results are presented in Fig. 6.13. The resulting figures show that as with the earlier case, weak supervision helps in improving the performance of the learning algorithm. We get a jump start and a steeper learning curve in this case as well. Again, the results are statistically significant for small number of gold standard examples. Both experiments conclusively prove that adding probabilistic examples as weak supervision enables our learning algorithm to improve upon its performance in the presence of small number of gold standard data thus validating the hypothesis that world knowledge helps when manual annotations are expensive.

6.5 Discussion and Wrap-Up

In this book, we presented the first-of-its-kind learning algorithm for SRL models based on functional gradient boosting. The key idea is to consider learning as a series of regression models in a stage-wise manner. The advantage of this approach is that

---

[6] http://www.nfl.com.

[7] http://www.premierleague.com.

we can learn the structure of the models and their parameters simultaneously. We showed how to adapt this algorithm for learning multiple relational models—RDNs, MLNs, relational policies via imitation learning and even transfer learning. We also extended the algorithm to learn faithfully in the presence of missing data without making assumptions about the data. Finally, we demonstrated across several tasks including few different health care prediction problems, natural language processing tasks, transfer learning in relational domains etc. The variety of applications clearly show demonstrate the broad applicability and usefulness of the boosting approach to learning in relational problems.

Following this work, there are some interesting future research directions: learning acyclic directed models still remains an interesting future direction. One of the key bottlenecks to learning these directed models is checking for acyclicity in the ground network. This is a costly operation that needs to be sped up for large tasks. Determining how to leverage the power of boosting without expensively checking for such cycles remains a challenge. Another direction is to leverage the recent successes in probabilistic data bases (Niu et al. 2012) to accelerate learning SRL models. Most of the SRL models appear to learn mainly horn clauses and such clauses can be learned faster using data base concepts. Scaling this up is certainly a promising direction. Finally, combining the recent results in lifted inference to better integrate learning and inference remains an interesting direction for future research.

Appendix A
BooSTR System

Our code base for Boosted STatistical Relational learning (BooSTR) is available at `http://pages.cs.wisc.edu/~tushar/Boostr/index.html`. We present a brief documentation about how to run our code here, which is also available on our webpage.

A.1 Commandline Arguments

A.1.1 General Arguments

-l : Use this flag, if you want to enable learning.

-i : Use this flag, if you want to enable inference.

-noBoost : Use this flag, if you dont want to use Boosting.

-train <Training directory> : Path to the training directory in WILL format.

-test <Testing directory> : Path to the testing directory in WILL format.

-model <Model directory> : Path to the directory with the stored models[or where they will be stored]. Default location: "Training directory"/models

-target <target predicates> : Comma separated list of predicates that need to be learned/inferred.

-trees <Number of trees>: Number of Boosting trees. Default: 20. Ignored if noBoost is set.

© The Author(s) 2014
S. Natarajan et al., *Boosted Statistical Relational Learners*,
SpringerBriefs in Computer Science, DOI 10.1007/978-3-319-13644-8

-step <Step Length>: Default step length for functional gradient. Default: 1.

-modelSuffix <suffix>: All the trees/models are saved with this suffix appended to the filenames.

-aucJarPath <path to auc.jar> If this is not set correctly, AUC values are not computed.

-testNegPosRatio <Negative/Positive ratio>: Ratio of negatives to positive for testing. Default: 2. Set to −1 to disable sampling.

A.1.2 MLN Arguments

-mln : Set this flag, if you want to learn MLNs instead of RDNs
-mlnClause : Set this flag, if you want to learn MLNs via clausal representation. If not set, the tree representation will be used.
-numMLNClause : If -mlnclause is set, set the number of clauses learned during each gradient step.
-mlnClauseLen : If -mlnclause is set, set the length of the clauses learned during each gradient step.

A.2   Sample Scripts

```
!#\bin\bash
java -cp ../WILL.jar edu.wisc.cs.Boosting.RDN.RunBoostedRDN \
  -aucJarPath ".." \
  -target cancer \
  -trees 20 \
  -l -train ../data/toy_cancer/train/

!#\bin\bash
java -cp ../WILL.jar edu.wisc.cs.Boosting.RDN.RunBoostedRDN \
-aucJarPath ".." \
-target cancer \
-trees 20 \
-model ../data/toy_cancer/train/models \
-i -test ../data/toy_cancer/test/
```

References

Biba M, Ferilli S, Esposito F (2008) Structure learning of Markov logic networks through iterated local search. In: ECAI

Bilenko M, Mooney R (2003) Adaptive duplicate detection using learnable string similarity measures. In: KDD

Bishop C (2006) Pattern Recognition and Machine Learning. Springer-Verlag New York, Inc.

Blockeel H, Raedt LD (1998) Top-down induction of first-order logical decision trees. Artificial Intelligence 101:285–297

Chambers N, Jurafsky D (2008) Jointly combining implicit constraints improves temporal ordering. In: EMNLP

Chickering D (1996) Learning Bayesian networks is NP-Complete. In: Learning from Data: Artificial Intelligence and Statistics V, Springer-Verlag, pp 121–130

Craven M, Kumlien J (1999) Constructing biological knowledge bases by extracting information from text sources. In: ISMB

Craven M, Shavlik J (1996) Extracting tree-structured representations of trained networks. In: NIPS

Cristianini N, Shawe-Taylor J (2000) An Introduction to Support Vector Machines and Other Kernel-based Learning Methods. Cambridge University Press

Davis J, Goadrich M (2006) The relationship between Precision-Recall and ROC curves. In: ICML

de Salvo Braz R Amir E Roth D (2005) Lifted first order probabilistic inference. In: IJCAI

Dempster A, Laird N, Rubin D (1977) Maximum likelihood from incomplete data via the EM algorithm. Journal of the Royal Statistical Society B.39:1–38

Devlin S, Kudenko D, Grzes M (2011) An empirical study of potential-based reward shaping and advice in complex, multi-agent systems. Advances in Complex Systems 14(2):251–278

Dietterich T, Ashenfelter A, Bulatov Y (2004) Training conditional random fields via gradient tree boosting. In: ICML

Domingos P, Lowd D (2009) Markov Logic: An Interface Layer for AI. Morgan & Claypool

Freund Y, Schapire R (1996) Experiments with a new boosting algorithm. In: ICML

Friedman J (2001) Greedy function approximation: A gradient boosting machine. Annals of Statistics pp 1189–1232

Friedman N (1998) The Bayesian structural EM algorithm. In: UAI

Getoor L, Taskar B (eds) (2007) Introduction to Statistical Relational Learning. MIT Press

Getoor L, Friedman N, Koller D, Pfeffer A (2001) Learning probabilistic relational models. Relational Data Mining pp 307–338

Gutmann B, Kersting K (2006) TildeCRF: Conditional random fields for logical sequences. In: ECML

Heckerman D, Chickering D, Meek C, Rounthwaite R, Kadie C (2001) Dependency networks for inference, collaborative filtering, and data visualization. Journal of Machine Learning Research 1:49–75

© The Author(s) 2014

S. Natarajan et al., *Boosted Statistical Relational Learners*,

SpringerBriefs in Computer Science, DOI 10.1007/978-3-319-13644-8

Heckerman D, Meek C, Koller D (2004) Probabilistic models for relational data. Tech. Rep. MSR-TR-2004-30

Hoffmann R, Zhang C, Ling X, Zettlemoyer L, Weld DS (2011) Knowledge-based weak supervision for information extraction of overlapping relations. In: ACL

Huynh T, Mooney R (2009) Max-margin weight learning for markov logic networks. In: ECML/PKDD

Huynh T, Mooney R (2011) Online max-margin weight learning for markov logic networks. In: SDM

Jaeger M (1997) Relational Bayesian networks. In: UAI

Jaeger M (2007) Parameter learning for relational Bayesian networks. In: ICML

John G, Langley P (1995) Estimating continuous distributions in bayesian classifiers. In: Eleventh Conference on Uncertainty in Artificial Intelligence, Morgan Kaufmann, pp 338–345

Kameya Y, Sato T (2000) Efficient EM learning with tabulation for parameterized logic programs. In: Computational Logic

Kersting K (2012) Lifted probabilistic inference. In: ECAI 2012 - 20th European Conference on Artificial Intelligence. Including Prestigious Applications of Artificial Intelligence (PAIS-2012) System Demonstrations Track, Montpellier, France, August 27–31, 2012, pp 33–38

Kersting K, De Raedt L (2007) Bayesian logic programming: Theory and tool. In: Getoor L, Taskar B (eds) An Introduction to Statistical Relational Learning

Kersting K, Driessens K (2008) Non-parametric policy gradients: A unified treatment of propositional and relational domains. In: ICML

Kersting K, Raiko T (2005) 'Say EM' for selecting probabilistic models for logical sequences. In: UAI

Kersting K, Ahmadi B, Natarajan S (2009) Counting Belief Propagation. In: UAI

Khot T, Natarajan S, Kersting K, Shavlik J (2011) Learning Markov logic networks via functional gradient boosting. In: ICDM

Khot T, Srivastave S, Natarajan S, Shavlik J (2012) Learning relational structure for temporal relation extraction. In: StarAI Workshop in UAI

Khot T, Natarajan S, Kersting K, Shavlik J (2014) Gradient-based boosting for statistical relational learning : The Markov logic network and missing data cases. Machine Learning Under review

Kindermann R, Snell J (1980) Markov Random Fields and Their Applications. American Mathematical Society

Kok S, Domingos P (2005) Learning the structure of Markov logic networks. In: ICML

Kok S, Domingos P (2009) Learning Markov logic network structure via hypergraph lifting. In: ICML

Kok S, Domingos P (2010) Learning Markov logic networks using structural motifs. In: ICML

Kok S, Sumner M, Richardson M, Singla P, Poon H, Lowd D, Wang J, Nath A, Domingos P (2010) The Alchemy system for statistical relational AI. Tech. rep., Department of Computer Science and Engineering, University of Washington, Seattle, WA. http://alchemy.cs.washington.edu.

Koller D, Friedman N (2009) Probabilistic Graphical Models: Principles and Techniques. The MIT Press

Kuhlmann G, Stone P, Mooney RJ, Shavlik JW (2004) Guiding a reinforcement learner with natural language advice: Initial results in robocup soccer. In: AAAI Workshop on Supervisory Control of Learning and Adaptive Systems

Lavrac N, Dzeroski S (1994) Inductive logic programming - techniques and applications. Ellis Horwood series in artificial intelligence, Ellis Horwood

Li X, Zhou Z (2007) Structure learning of probabilistic relational models from incomplete relational data. In: ECML

Lowd D, Davis J (2010) Learning Markov network structure with decision trees. In: ICDM

Lowd D, Domingos P (2007) Efficient weight learning for markov logic networks. In: PKDD

McCarty CA, Wilke RA, Giampietro PF, Wesbrook SD, Caldwell MD (2005) Marshfield clinic personalized medicine research project (pmrp): design, methods and recruitment for a large population-based biobank. Personalized Medicine 2(1):49–79

McCarty CA, Peissig P, Caldwell MD, Wilke RA (2008) The marshfield clinic personalized medicine research project: 2008 scientific update and lessons learned in the first 6 years. Personalized Medicine 5(5):529–542

Mihalkova L, Mooney R (2007) Bottom-up learning of Markov logic network structure. In: ICML

Milch B, Marthi B, Russell S (2004) BLOG: Relational modeling with unknown objects. In: Proceedings of the SRL Workshop in ICML

Mintz M, Bills S, Snow R, Jurafsky D (2009) Distant supervision for relation extraction without labeled data. In: ACL

Mitchell T (1997) Machine Learning. McGraw-Hill, Inc.

Muggleton S, Raedt LD (1994) Inductive logic programming: Theory and methods. Journal of Logic Programming 19/20:629–679

Natarajan S, Tadepalli P, Altendorf E, Dieterich TG, Fern A, Restificar A (2005) Learning first-order probabilistic models with combining rules. In: Proceedings of the International Conference in Machine Learning

Natarajan S, Tadepalli P, Dieterich T, Fern A (2008) Learning first-order probabilistic models with combining rules. Annals of Mathematics and AI 54(1–3):223–256

Natarajan S, Joshi S, Tadepalli P, Kristian K, Shavlik J (2011) Imitation learning in relational domains: A functional-gradient boosting approach. In: IJCAI

Natarajan S, Joshi S, Saha B, Edwards A, E Moody TK, Kersting K, Whitlow C, Maldjian J (2012a) A machine learning pipeline for three-way classification of alzheimer patients from structural magnetic resonance images of the brain. In: IEEE Conference on Machine Learning and Applications (ICMLA)

Natarajan S, Khot T, Kersting K, Guttmann B, Shavlik J (2012b) Gradient-based boosting for statistical relational learning: The relational dependency network case. Machine Learning

Natarajan S, Joshi S, Saha B, Edwards A, E Moody TK, Kersting K, Whitlow C, Maldjian J (2013a) Relational learning helps in three-way classification of alzheimer patients from structural magnetic resonance images of the brain. International Journal of Machine Learning and Cybernetics

Natarajan S, Kersting K, Ip E, Jacobs D, Carr J (2013b) Early prediction of coronary artery calcification levels using machine learning. In: Innovative Applications in AI

Neville J, Jensen D (2007) Relational dependency networks. In: Getoor L, Taskar B (eds) Introduction to Statistical Relational Learning, MIT Press, pp 653–692

Neville J, Jensen D, Friedland L, Hay M (2003a) Learning relational probability trees. In: KDD

Neville J, Jensen D, Gallagher B (2003b) Simple estimators for relational bayesian classifiers. In: ICDM

Ngo L, Haddawy P (1995) Probabilistic Logic programming and Bayesian networks. In: ACSC

Nilsson N (1986) Probabilistic logic. Artificial Intelligence 28(1):71–88

Niu F, Zhang C, Ré C, Shavlik J (2012) Elementary: Large-scale knowledge-base construction via machine learning and statistical inference. IJSWIS Special Issue on Web-Scale Knowledge Extraction

Pearl J (1988) Probabilistic Reasoning in Intelligent Systems: Networks of Plausible Inference. Morgan Kaufmann Publishers Inc.

Poole D (1993) Probabilistic Horn abduction and Bayesian networks. AIJ pp 81–129

Poole D (2003) First-Order probabilistic inference. In: IJCAI

Poon H, Domingos P (2007) Joint inference in information extraction. In: AAAI, pp 913–918

Quinlan J (1993) C4.5: programs for machine learning

Quinlan JR (1996) Bagging, boosting, and c4.5. In: AAAI/IAAI, Vol. 1, pp 725–730

Raedt LD (2008) Logical and Relational Learning: From ILP to MRDM (Cognitive Technologies). Springer-Verlag New York, Inc.

Richardson M, Domingos P (2004) Markov logic networks. Tech. rep., Department of Computer Science and Engineering, University of Washington, Seattle, WA. http://www.cs.washington.edu/homes/pedrod/mln.pdf.

Richardson M, Domingos P (2006) Markov logic networks. Machine Learning 62:107–136

Riedel S, Yao L, McCallum A (2010) Modeling relations and their mentions without labeled text. In: ECML PKDD

Russell S, Norvig P (2003) Artificial Intelligence: A Modern Approach. Pearson Education

Sato T, Kameya Y (2001) Parameter learning of logic programs for symbolic-statistical modeling. Journal of Artificial Intelligence Research pp 391–454

Shavlik J, Natarajan S (2009) Speeding up inference in Markov logic networks by preprocessing to reduce the size of the resulting grounded network. In: IJCAI

Singla P, Domingos P (2005) Discriminative training of Markov logic networks. In: AAAI

Singla P, Domingos P (2006) Entity resolution with Markov logic. In: ICDM, pp 572–582

Singla P, Domingos P (2008) Lifted first-order belief propagation. In: AAAI

Stone P, Sutton R (2001) Scaling reinforcement learning toward RoboCup soccer. In: ICML

Takamatsu S, Sato I, Nakagawa H (2012) Reducing wrong labels in distant supervision for relation extraction. In: ACL

Taskar B, Abeel P, Koller D (2002) Discriminative probabilistic models for relational data. In: UAI

Torrey L, Shavlik J, Walker T, Maclin R (2007) Relational macros for transfer in reinforcement learning. In: ILP

Torrey L, Shavlik J, Walker T, Maclin R (2010) Transfer learning via advice taking. In: Advances in Machine Learning I, pp 147–170

UzZaman N, Allen JF (2010) TRIPS and TRIOS system for TempEval-2: Extracting temporal information from text. In: SemEval

Van Laer W Dehaspe L De Raedt L (1994) Applications of a logical discovery engine. In: WKDD

Verhagen M, Gaizauskas R, Schilder F, Hepple M, Katz G, Pustejovsky J (2007) SemEval-2007 task 15: TempEval temporal relation identification. In: SemEval

Wei G, Tanner M (1990) A Monte Carlo implementation of the EM algorithm and the poor man's data augmentation algorithms. Journal of the American Statistical Association 85(411)

Weiss J, Natarajan S, Peissig P, McCarty C, Page D (2012a) Statistical relational learning to predict primary myocardial infarction from electronic health records. In: Innovative Applications in AI

Weiss J, Natarajan S, Peissig P, McCarty C, Page D (2012b) Statistical relational learning to predict primary myocardial infarction from electronic health records. In: AI Magazine

Yoshikawa K, Riedel S, Asahara M, Matsumoto Y (2009) Jointly identifying temporal relations with Markov Logic. In: ACL